The Stoic Body

An Ancient Twist to Modern Health

Philip Ghezelbash

Disclaimer:

These opinions and suggestions reflect the research and ideas of the author and aren't intended to substitute for services by a medical professional. All content here is for informational purposes only and should not be taken as medical advice. The author disclaims any responsibility for any adverse effects results from information in this book.

Philip's Disclaimer:

Don't do anything dumb. Treat this book as one of many sources of information and make grounded judgements. Use your common sense!

Always consult a doctor and/or a specialist before doing anything .

ISBN: 978-0473418465

A catalogue record for this book is available from the National Library of New Zealand.

Edited by Anne-Marie Emerson McDonald

Illustration by Bradley Smit

youtube.com/c/philipghezelbash

philipghezelbash.com

"The beginning and foundation of temperance lies in self-control in eating and drinking."

— Musonius Rufus

CONTENTS

PROLOGUE

This book is about Stoicism, a philosophy founded by Zeno of Citium. This book is also about modern health, fat loss and the general state of obesity in our society. Essentially, *The Stoic Body* is about using Stoicism as a foundation for the pursuit of good health.

In the prologue and introduction I will speak about some of the fundamental aspects of Stoic philosophy you need to know, and various other ideas about health in the modern world. Then I'll cover nutrition, fitness, psychology and how philosophy intertwines with them.

A quick note on gender: this book is written with a narrative directed towards men. Why? Because the ideal of Stoicism itself was masculine. However, this does not mean that women cannot be Stoics themselves, and there were classical Stoics who agreed with this.

In 301 BC Zeno developed Stoicism as he walked up and down under the colonnades of the *Stoa Poikile*, or Painted Porch, in Athens, and the Stoic school was established there. As the philosophy expanded and developed through Zeno's successors, Stoicism grew into the most influential Hellenistic philosophy of its time. The eventual decline of Stoicism came during the Roman Empire in AD 300. Very few formal philosophical writings from the classical Stoics actually survived – approximately 1 per cent – and most of Stoicism today is founded upon the reconstruction of a fraction of the original knowledge.

To the Stoics, the goal of man was not to shape the world, but instead to shape the will and the ability of man to adapt to a reality which is often out of our control and subject to fate. Stoicism produced men of immense will and discipline, and gave rise to individuals who would *do* rather than *think*. Stoicism was not about philosophy; it was about living philosophically.

Ethics in Stoicism is the effort, while logic and physics support the study of ethics. These are called the three *topoi*. Think of logic (reasoning about the world) as a sort of defence, and physics (the study of the world logic defends) as providing knowledge and proof. Ethics is then the fruit, the occurrence, essentially the result of reasoning about the world and gaining knowledge from it.

A *sophos* (sage) in classical philosophy is an individual who has perfect wisdom. In the context of Stoicism it is *almost* impossible for a mortal to become a sage. The sage is a moral ideal in which virtue (moral excellence) defines progression towards the ideal, a journey referred to as *prokopê* (making progress). Stoicism is a dualistic view of the intersection of the physical and spiritual manifestations of the universe. Today, the philosophy continues to teach us that there's a small part of the cosmos within us all. The best way to live according to the Stoics is to make decisions through virtue; it's in our best interests to live a life "in accordance with nature", as the Stoic motto says.

The more I've learned about the Stoics, the more I have found myself more drawn to the philosophy. What I've learned has helped me understand why it was one of the most respected schools of thought in the classical world, and more importantly, why it transcended through time, remaining so relevant in changing societies and culture. As I go deeper into Stoicism, more puzzle pieces, you could say, seem to be fitting into place in my life. In my pre-Stoic days the puzzle pieces seemed to be getting lost, and my memory of what the puzzle was supposed to look like began to fade.

As with many other individuals attracted to the philosophy, I feel compelled to share the wisdom, but I choose to do this through my own expertise, adding an ancient twist to health in the modern world, instead of simply paraphrasing repeated concepts. In recent years it would appear Stoicism has been having a cultural revival. I believe this movement has potential to grow if the philosophy is intertwined into other industries; in this case, health and well-being.

The wisdom of the Stoics can be applied to health, entrepreneurship and even dating, for the simple reason that the framework is based on human nature. The Stoics believed we are social animals. When you benefit others you benefit yourself; hence when you benefit your own health it will benefit the world and eventually come back to you.

Minus flying cars and travelling at the speed of light, cutting-edge technology today was science fiction merely a few decades ago. We now understand almost all there is to know about the human body down to a molecular level – yet obesity and lifestyle-related disease are our greatest opponents. In an age which dismisses much of ancient literature as old and outdated, more people are coming to realise that time must be taken to reflect on the wisdom of those who came before us in order to resolve of the issues in front of us. Many of our revolutionary ideas which seem so contemporary are based on the genius that preceded today's civilisation. We are the tree and the ancients are the roots; for a tree to grow its roots must be watered. We study the ancients because they were remarkably attuned to the nature of human psychology, which hasn't changed much.

In *The Stoic Body* you will be exposed to the teachings of some of the greatest classical Stoics – Epictetus, the Roman slave; Lucius Annaeus Seneca, the Roman dramatist and thinker; Zeno of Citium, the founder, teacher and scholar; Marcus Aurelius, the Roman military leader; and Gaius Musonius Rufus, the Roman knight. If it weren't for modern Stoic thinkers such as William Irvine, Donald Robertson, Ryan Holiday, William

Ferraiolo, Massimo Pigliucci, and many more, few outside of academia would be aware of this classical wisdom. With inspiration from these ancient and modern thinkers, and the latest in scientific research, comes a book which I envision adding a well overdue ancient twist to today's obesity epidemic.

If you're here for a science book, return it; if you're here for a work of philosophy, again, return the book. However, if you're here to explore how both fields intertwine and complement one another, then look no further.

INTRODUCTION

"Besides, it is a disgrace to grow old through
sheer carelessness before seeing what manner
of man you may become by developing your
bodily strength and beauty to their highest limit.
But you cannot see that, if you are careless; for
it will not come of its own accord."

– Socrates

Zeno of Citium (334–262 BC) was the founder of the
Stoic school of philosophy. According to Diogenes
Laërtius (AD 180–240) a biographer of Greek philoso-
phers, Zeno was a merchant, a tanned and haggard man, who
lived with few belongings. He was known as a temperate man.
(Little is known about Diogenes. He is mostly recognised as
a biographer of philosophers through his surviving work,
Lives and Opinions of Eminent Philosophers.) Diogenes describes
a legend in which Zeno stumbled upon a bookstore, where he
found himself drawn to Xenophon's writings about Socrates.
Xenophon (430–354 BC) is often credited as the authority on
Socrates. Socrates (470/469–399 BC), for those of you unaware,
was a classical Greek philosopher who is often recognised as
one of the founding fathers of Western philosophy. He was an
oracular and enigmatic figure who was sentenced to death by
drinking poison.

When Zeno came to Athens, the city was dominated by the doctrine of Socrates. As Zeno ventured to Athens from Cyprus in 300 BC, the *Stoa Poikile* (a pathway in the *agora*, or marketplace, of Athens) became a location he was fond of and attracted to. This location became the spot he would repeatedly use to teach and interact with his followers. The English word *stoic* originates from the Greek word *stōïkos*, translating to *portico* (covered walkway); hence the name of the philosophy.

From the very beginning, Stoicism was a Socratic philosophy. Cynicism, too, had a strong influence on Stoicism, as the Cynic philosopher Crates of Thebes (385–285 BC) taught Zeno. Zeno's development of Stoic philosophy was clearly based on the Socratic inspiration of virtue being the chief good, but also considered the accounts of Stilpo (whose ethical teachings influenced Pyrrho, the founder of Pyrrhonism). Stilpo would say that nothing of the external can be good or bad. The framework of Stoicism as a Socratic philosophy, along with influences such as Stilpo, essentially formed the unique Stoic ideal which separates it from other schools. This Stoic ideal holds that external goods are of indifferent value and ethically neutral, but still objects of desire we may long to pursue.

Physical strength and beauty was held in high regard in ancient Greece. It was commonplace for Greek males to be athletic and strong in their youth. Yet Socrates never went into detail when discussing physical matters. Instead we are left with fragments of his verbal accounts where he recognises that a man must be strong and in good health; however, this was highly superficial to him. For someone who is educated or is seeking to become educated, physical strength can *never* rival the merit of practising reason and debate. To Socrates, a man's true strength and character will never be revealed by the size of his biceps or the capacity of his lungs, but only through his thirst for knowledge. This is a good time for you to think about your own intentions for wishing to improve your health. Ask yourself: "Is my desire out of vanity, to banish insecurity, or is it for the pursuit of something deeper?"

The attitude of Socrates aligns itself well with the Stoic duality between the body and the mind. Socrates was known for his protruding belly and unbalanced physical attributes. What many don't know is that he was a decorated military hero. Some scholars believe that his heroic acts at the Battle of Delium (424 BC) brought him to fame in Athens. Despite his physical looks in his later years, his pupils still saw him as a beautiful man, but *not* for his physical appearance. Socrates was beautiful to his pupils because of his penetrating intellect.

For the Stoics, the cosmos is a whole and single entity. A living organism, you could say, that is held together through pneuma, the "breath of life". The world for the Stoic is a very carefully crafted and rational system. Anything that seems bad, such as poor health or "unfair" circumstances, is attributed to the holistic reasoning of the universe, the impersonal god. Whatever seems unfortunate right now is simply proven to be for the higher good, over time.

Zeno of Citium explained virtue as "living consistently", while Cleanthes (330–230 BC) added the clause "with nature". The Stoic motto was to live life "in accordance with nature" as a whole; to be as one with the cosmos through motives and actions. Virtue (moral excellence) is the vessel to living the good life. Since virtue is the only true good, naturally it becomes necessary.

The detailed taxonomy of virtue for the Stoics is divided into four types: wisdom (*sophia*), courage (*andreia*), justice (*dikaiosyne*) and temperance (*sophrosyne*). Living through moral goodness frees us from our attachments, dependencies, passions and ideals. Being virtuous can be described as pure rationality with ourselves; what virtue *isn't* is a quality that we magically possesses. Virtue is earned through overcoming challenges. By intentionally exposing ourselves to them and exploring dilemmas and tribulations, we bring forth this innate spark of rationality we were all born with. These experiences open the opportunity for virtue to "take place" through adopting the appropriate frame of equanimity and control over one's actions, in response to divine interventions.

The opposite of virtue is vice. Vice can be described as incorrect value judgements, which are not made by rational beings. It is also divided into four types: foolishness, injustice, cowardice and intemperance.

The Stoics who came after Zeno disagree on a number of issues, such as sex and even the consumption of meat (as we'll cover in detail later on). Perhaps the most important disagreement is the dispute between Cleanthes and Chrysippus about the bond of the different virtues. Zeno speaks about each individual virtue being its own kind of wisdom; while Cleanthes asserts all virtues are one: wisdom. Chrysippus tells us that each virtue is one of its own, a "niche" of wisdom – a coexisting and pluralistic ideology.

In the Western world today, obesity remains more abundant than ever, despite objective knowledge of the advantages of good health. The sheer amount of food consumed in the Western world has become as harmful as the lack of it in developing countries. As scientific research continues to expand, we are becoming more aware that many of our issues regarding obesity and poor health are deeply embedded in our survival instincts. Today we live in a privileged world. The commodity of food has become something of little value. Food has become a *right* rather than a *privilege*.

Imagine our bodies as the foundation of our homes and our intellect as the house itself. Despite the importance of the house itself we cannot build it without the foundation, and so it makes sense to build the structural integrity of the foundation to the best of our ability. If the foundation is strong and stable, then the house is able to withstand the inevitable earthquakes, storms and fires of life.

How often have we received opportunities from the world and denied them? How often have we failed to seize a worthy opportunity? There is only a limited time fixed for each of us, and if we do not use this time wisely to clear the clouds from our minds, then our minds will simply go and never return. If you believe without a doubt that something is too difficult for you to accomplish on your own, I would argue this is not based on a reasonable estimation, but rather on your *perception* of it. Do not make the mistake of thinking a goal is impossible for you. If losing weight after years of obesity was done by another and this was comfortable to the nature of who he was, then be sure that any achievement with parallel or even greater difficulty is a possibility for you too.

The definition of the word *diet* has been warped and aligned into the sphere of the transformative, the dramatic and the very dangerous implication that shocking and immediate change is a positive outcome. Increasingly more trainers, dieticians, nutritionists and psychologists are staying away from this term because of the perception it may frame about what truly matters in the pursuit of health. The issue I have with this type of change is that it cannot be maintained. Progress depends on whether an individual is consistent, and this is reliant on whether a programme is sustainable. What this means is that no matter how "incredible" or even scientifically correct a diet or workout programme is, it can never be ideal if there is no consistency and repetition.

This is where philosophy becomes relevant. You must understand that you are not here to necessarily lose fat, but to improve what you can control – your self-discipline and character. The reason I have written an entire book around Stoicism and health is because virtue is often expressed as a by-product of the activities which precede a strong, healthy and athletic body. As with Socrates' position, the Stoics understood that health remains irrelevant to the wider picture of true happiness. No health is guaranteed, no body is guaranteed, *ever*. No matter how perfect a specific programme or method is, there is no reasonable way to secure its benefits. Your testosterone will fall, you will age, your skin will sag; but your self-discipline and temperance, which is worthy of praise, is under your control and will last a lifetime.

Epigenetics translates to "upon the gene". We now know conclusively that our genes react to our behaviour. The way we act, behave and how we think directly affects how our genes express themselves. Researcher Catherine Shanahan rather frighteningly points out that these gene expressions carry through to the next generation. According to a 2003 study from *Molecular and Cellular Biology*, laboratory mice fed with specific vitamin blends show correlated features – such as weight and susceptibilities to certain ailments and behaviours – in successive generations. Some very interesting research led by Brian Dias at Emory University School of Medicine tells us that mice whose father or grandfather learned to associate the smell of cherry blossom with an electric shock became more jumpy in the presence of the same odour, and responded to lower concentrations of it than normal mice.

Health and fitness is usually pertained as a selfish act, one which the media has often portrayed as one of narcissism. But if we look deeper and examine the genetic changes good health provokes, then we see that the decisions we make today affect not only the environment, not only the greater good of our community due to happiness and mortality rates, it will also – through direct epigenetic inheritance – influence much of the genetic kick-start our children receive. The Stoics emphasise that we have ethical obligations to our wider community, especially as we age, so why would health be an exception?

The irony of technological development is that as the internet and the abundance of accessible information grows, it becomes extremely difficult to pinpoint exactly what the precise cause and treatment of an ailment is. A quick search on Google may give you advice on how to drop weight in a way which your doctor never mentioned once. Surely Google cannot account for years of a practitioner's medical training – or can it? Yes, it's also naive to say that we shouldn't take advantage of this information. The best scenario is a balanced respect for both sources, as regressing back to an age where the only treatments were those available from just one practitioner is clearly not a good idea. We are constantly bombarded with new information. It is not my intention to bombard you with more and outline a new revolutionary step-by-step method to achieving any specific health-related goal.

The Stoic Body is about providing you with concepts, ideas, information backed by science and, most critically, a framework which you can work from. I want you to finish this book and know without a doubt that you are able to dissect through the gimmicks and the countless marketing schemes to come to reasoned and well-informed decisions in regard to your health and well-being, comfortable and confident in making the right decisions. *The Stoic Body* will teach you how to overcome your evolutionary programming which in today's world has normalised a pleasure-seeking lifestyle. Today we seem to move through life in search of our next pleasure, but in doing so we are running away from what truly gives us peace of mind. The right pursuit is often more difficult and so the majority make the conscious decision to recline into their "evolutionary autopilot", as Stoic philosopher William Irvine phrased it. Here you will learn how to revoke the compulsive force that pulls you out of a congruent, tempered and disciplined path. With careful consideration of the following ideas I am confident that you will take away some important lessons which you can apply from the moment you read them.

As Irvine did in his book *A Guide to the Good Life,* I am attempting to develop a "brand" of Stoicism. *The Stoic Body* reflects how I apply the philosophy to my own aptitudes and my own position in life. If this book ends up not being your cup of tea, so be it. You will be glad to know that there are many other "brands" of the philosophy, both classical and modern, with one surely fitting your taste.

PART ONE:
DEFINING NATURE

"Our motto, as you know, is 'live according to nature'; but it is quite contrary to nature to torture the body, to hate unlaboured elegance, to be dirty on purpose, to eat food that is not only plain, but disgusting and forbidding."

– Seneca

THE HIGH PRIESTESS

Marcus Aurelius (AD 121–180), known as the last of the "five good emperors", was the Emperor of Rome from AD 161 to 180. He is a large source of our modern understanding of Stoic philosophy. His book *Meditations* (literally, "[that which is] to himself"), is a series of personal notes and ideas on Stoicism which many consider one of the greatest works the world has ever seen.

Marcus Aurelius said, "You will give yourself peace if you do every act of your life as if it were the last." This quotation made me realise that if we are to live "according to nature", we must first accept that nature takes life erratically and holds no concern for circumstances or what is fair. When you become aware of your poor decisions or are in midst of a decision, remind yourself that your actions must always emulate the urgency of a man whose forthcoming death has been revealed.

So what does it mean to truly live "according to nature"? The word *nature* began in Greek as *physis*. *Physis* describes nature's constant change and adaption into various archetypes. We each have a specific genetic structure, predetermined by our parents and ancestral lineage. What is indisputable is that we lack *some* free will, as we are governed by forces outside our control. We are born with a predisposition to look and act in a certain manner. We have no choice whether we are born in 1489 or 1984; time will never be in our control. The era that we are born in dictates the framework of reality we experience. We often follow a path aligned with a societal narrative of some sort, assigned to us from a young age, and we mirror our actions through comparison to the behaviour of others. We have a deep longing to belong, to experience the unity of bonds and friendship. Often this deep desire is what leads to problems. We must remember to constantly question ourselves, asking: "Is the way I'm living the *right* way?" We do this in order to distinguish what is *influenced* and what is *natural*.

Lucius Annaeus Seneca (4 BC–AD 65) was a Roman Stoic philosopher, dramatist, the tutor of Nero and a strong influence on William Shakespeare. Seneca tells us that to some extent we cannot live according to nature without athleticism and good health. Not caring about our health places at risk the joy we are capable of experiencing. To counter his opinion, we could say, "Who are you to claim that a lack of health cannot be a defining reflection of nature itself?"

This is precisely what the German philosopher Friedrich Wilhelm Nietzsche (1844–1900) would argue many centuries later. Nietzsche wrote about poetry and cultural criticisms, and had a fondness for aphorism and irony. He is well known for his work on the doctrines of Eternal Recurrence and *Übermensch* (in English, Superman). Later in his life he became fascinated in cultivating methods which would eventually be used to overcome cultural, social and moral contexts in the pursuit of new values. In his work *Beyond Good and Evil* Nietzsche criticised the Stoic motto of "living according to nature" in this way:

"You desire to LIVE 'according to Nature'? Oh, you noble Stoics, what fraud of words! Imagine to yourselves a being like Nature, boundlessly extravagant, boundlessly indifferent, without purpose or consideration, without pity or justice, at once fruitful and barren and uncertain: imagine to yourselves INDIFFERENCE as a power – how COULD you live in accordance with such indifference?

"To live – is not that just endeavouring to be otherwise than this Nature? Is not living valuing, preferring, being unjust, being limited, endeavouring to be different? And granted that your imperative, 'living according to Nature', means actually the same as 'living according to life' – how could you do DIFFERENTLY? Why should you make a principle out of what you yourselves are, and must be?"

In a conversation with a friend I was presented by an argument similar to the premise of Nietzsche but phrased in the context of this book's subject. For a moment imagine yourself transported to the jungles of Papua New Guinea...

Picture a tribe that has never been in contact with the outside world. They are a very spiritual tribe. As part of their metaphysical framework, they have several priestesses. The high priestess, as part of a ritual in which the entire tribe takes part, assumes the role of their tribal goddess. In this role, she is forced to eat vast quantities of food designated as a sacrifice for the goddess. The fatter this priestess becomes the more elated and ecstatic the tribe is. They are so happy. They believe that the fatness of their priestess equates to a happy goddess. You cannot say that the priestess's obesity is then a vice. *You cannot say that her fatness is unnatural.* The happiness and morale boost that her obesity brings to the tribe outweighs the damage it does to her body ten-fold. Is it still a vice?

So who are the Stoics to say that there is a way of doing nature *differently?*

Nietzsche's wording takes out the context of what living in accordance to nature *actually* means. Stoicism shows us that our suffering comes innately from what we *wish* to be different; suffering comes from our wish to change the unchangeable. When we wish nature to be different than it is, we suffer. It's not that nature itself is the cause of our suffering, rather it is our perspective on what nature "should be", rather than what it is.

Amor fati, often translated as "loving and accepting your fate", is Nietzsche's way of describing the attitude of how we should view everything that happens in our lives, even if that is suffering, loss or injury. *Amor fati* doesn't mean we need to improve our circumstances, because sometimes we can't improve the external, but rather – as Nietzsche's concept of Eternal Recurrence says – we should accept them so that no matter what we are exposed to, life can be lived at the same level of satisfaction.

Nietzsche's concept of *amor fati* has its roots in the *Enchiridion* of Epictetus. Epictetus (AD 50–135) was a Greek Stoic philosopher, born as a slave in modern-day Turkey. He told us: "Don't seek to have events happen as you wish, but wish them to happen as they do happen, and all will be well with you."

If living according to nature is reacting to life's objective suffering by being indifferent to it, is this not appropriating reason and rationality as the core of your being? Isn't this the very essence of living according to nature?

Nietzsche goes on to say: "But this is an old and everlasting story: what happened in old times with the Stoics still happens today, as soon as ever a philosophy begins to believe in itself. It always creates the world in its own image; it cannot do otherwise; philosophy is this tyrannical impulse itself, the most spiritual Will to Power, the will to 'creation of the world', the will to the *causa prima*."

If we look at his beliefs it becomes apparent that Nietzsche found Stoicism relatable. His views on Christianity formed out of an innate dissatisfaction with life and its unknown answers. Nietzsche famously tells us that "God is dead", which in itself aligns with Stoic belief in the sense that Stoicism encourages a man to be satisfied not with a promise for an afterlife, but through rational encounters with virtue. Nietzsche tells us that because God is in fact dead, Übermensch is the new creator of our values. These new values are not necessarily the same as our old ones; instead, our new love for life is created by the change in newly acquired archetypes of the human condition. Stoicism simply tells us that *this* is life and in order to do your best and live up to your potential you must act and live with virtue. There is no promise of the end of suffering. If suffering were to end or be a plausible outcome, sagehood and perfect wisdom would be a possibility.

Previously I touched upon the controversy surrounding whether a sage is actually a state one can achieve within the span of a lifetime. The Stoics had a saying that a sage is "as rare as the Ethiopian phoenix". This was a mythical bird which was born every five hundred years. There's some interesting dialogue between Epictetus and his pupils around being a sage, in which he asks them if any of them think he is a sage. His answer is that of course he isn't. Zeno never claimed to be a sage, and neither did any other of the classical scholars. This is fundamentally important in dissecting this problem.

In a conversation with author Donald Robertson, both he and I came to an agreement on the idea that one who claims being a sage must "continue to assume he's flawed", to quote Mr Robertson. Thus the claim – and elevation of one's identity to essentially being "perfect" – paradoxically may be used as evidence to counter the claim. The implication is that most fall within the unflattering category of the layman. Stoicism has a "band of brothers" sort of attitude, an air of "we're all in this together" – rather than some sort of competition to see who can become more perfect. At least, that's how I see it.

We are reminded by Stoicism that there is a dichotomy between our movement through the cosmos. We either have control or we don't have control. This belief system doesn't reinforce any higher desire to be rewarded for living well, but simply for the act of doing it. There is nothing more affirming and assuring than living for no reward. Doesn't Nietzsche tell us that we should love to be in existence, even if this existence brings suffering and pain?

Consider the following examples. Are they not the intentions of nature?

- When we are fit, our blood pressure is *stable*.
- When we weigh the appropriate weight, our heart pumps blood *optimally*.
- When we eat healthy food, our mind functions as it *should*.
- When we have a strong body the integrity of our bones is *solidified*.

We are *meant* to behave like this. But again you may question: "Who am I to say that our blood pressure being stable is how we are *meant* to live?" This is simply reaffirmed by increased chances for survival and longevity. It is not natural for us to decrease our chances of survival and of leaving behind our DNA by provoking ill health. But to have abnormal blood pressure does not exclude us from being natural beings; we are still part of the natural world, but if living unjustly, we are then simply categorised as beings in opposition to it. Seneca tells us: "Virtue is according to nature; vice is opposed to it and hostile." We live for our own self-preservation; if not, then there would be no point. But if there was in fact no point, then there would simply be a void between birth and death, not life itself!

To begin with, the Stoics recognised the above mentioned four cardinal virtues of wisdom, courage, justice and temperance; but also more specific ones within each of these acknowledged categories. An example is wisdom being inclusive of good judgement, resourcefulness; courage is divided into perseverance, confidence; justice as kindness, sociability. Temperance, most central to the body, is subdivided into seemliness, self-discipline, self-control and modesty.

The Stoics said that a stick is either straight or crooked, thus there is no in-between. You're either living justly or unjustly.

THE PHYSICAL SAGE

Human beings have an innate preference for beauty. It serves as a survival function. American maxillofacial surgeon Dr Stephen Marquardt created a mask to illustrate how the mathematical formula of phi (which defines the very healthy growth of plants and animals) can be applied to the face of human beings to help understand what these preferences of beauty are and how they are expressed universally. An example could be a wider jaw – a symbol of beauty, but also a sign of higher testosterone levels (libido, muscle mass, red blood cells and sperm) and allowing room for all teeth to fit (a narrow jaw can lead to wisdom teeth removal). Another is wider hips for females, symbolising fertility and youth. Health and beauty are extremely interlinked, more than we may wish to admit. Health increases beauty and intelligence; beauty and intelligence increase health.

Sagehood is the ideal for a Stoic, but this is impossible to achieve. Even if you disagree with this statement, the truth remains that most of us fall within an unflattering category. The same idea can be applied to the aesthetic of the body. The shape of the body can never be sculpted to be "perfect", not only on the account of individual genetic predisposition or subjectivity in beauty, but based on more ubiquitous grounds – we all die. We can parallel this "myth of perfection" to the physical issues of dysmorphia and dissatisfaction with one's body which are becoming increasingly common in a generation where gym culture has become heavily normalised and elevated as a requirement for the status of the self. *Adonis Complex* is the term used to describe the muscle dysmorphia affecting boys and men.

Adonis was a Greek mythological demi-god – half-man, half-god – who embodied and represented the perfect masculine ideal of beauty. His idealised figure was irresistible to the young women of ancient Greece. His figure was so gravitating that even Aphrodite, the goddess of love and pleasure, submitted to her lustful desire for Adonis. The Adonis Complex issue can be seen in every corner of our society (television, magazines and most importantly, the internet). This distortion portrays to the world an idealised version of the masculine self, which is impossible to achieve; yet it is portrayed to be a realistic accomplishment by marketers draining money from the pockets of the insecure. With this comes the psychological danger of people attaching intrinsic value and self-worth to the external.

This isn't a gender issue so I'm not proclaiming whether women or men face it more, although it's common knowledge that woman are faced with more pronounced aesthetic ideals. What I am saying is that men too face this issue and it is *different*, which makes it unnoticeable and potentially more dangerous. The Adonis Complex is an obsessional self-concern for one's physical appearance and, most harmful of all the underlying subconscious feelings, dissatisfaction and inadequacy, knowing that the individualised "physical sage" one has envisioned will never be achieved.

Imagine the Adonis Complex as a virus. This virus is contagious and has infected everybody who has been exposed to mainstream media. Despite the virus being in everybody's bloodstream it is occasionally inactive. When the virus does become active through weakening of the immune system (self-esteem), it spreads rapidly and can infect the entire body and mind.

Now perhaps it may seem like I am leaning towards

criticising the growing popularity of health and fitness, but this could not be further from the truth; I'm simply recognising the other side of the coin. (The general impact that the "gym revolution" has had on our society is useful; we have a problem and this popularisation acts as a solution.) With such dramatic increases in the popularity of a movement, another extreme is going to surface and it should not be ignored in discussion, as poor health of the body is not only about weight gain. Opposing extremes can be just as dangerous but more difficult to see since they are outside of the social narrative.

Muscle dysmorphia is the medical term for the Adonis Complex, but you may also have heard the term *bigorexia* (the antonym of anorexia). The basic idea of bigorexia is that a man will look at his reflection and see a body shape inferior to the standards ingrained in his subconscious. "I'm too skinny", "I'm weak", "I'm not a man because of the size of my muscles" – these are the obsessive thoughts of someone with bigorexia. To some, this may seem ridiculous, or it may seem all too familiar. The point is that this issue is *real* and it is growing. When the "virus" spreads, this dysmorphia exacerbates the rate at which the infected individual will injure and re-injure themselves.

If you are sitting at home and you are cold, you may possibly decide to light the fire. Why would you do this? To warm the house, obviously. After the fire is lit you may then decide that you are still too cold and you therefore you will choose to add more wood as the flame has nearly died out. Adding wood to the flame is not done with the intention of cooling the house – this would make no sense! Likewise, the intention of exercising and eating healthy in order to get a "six-pack" isn't done to provoke injury or ailments of any kind, as this too would be nonsensical. But sometimes we forget what type of wood we are placing into the fire. If we are in a rush to reignite a dying flame and aren't careful, we may mistake wet wood for dry wood, or we may place a large piece of wood in the fire instead of kindling — the flame could then die down and the house would eventually cool. The type of wood you use is analogous to your character and intent. Although wet wood may catch light the first time, or even the second and third, at some point the flame may burn out.

We must accept the fact, wholeheartedly, that you will *never* have 100 per cent control over your body. Epictetus makes it very clear what is within our control and what isn't: "Some things are within our power, while others are not. Within our power are opinion, motivation, desire, aversion, and, in a word, whatever is of our own doing; not within our power are our body, our property, reputation, office, and, in a word, whatever is not of our own doing." This is a fundamental idea of Stoicism, known as the Dichotomy of Control.

When you believe this, perfection becomes an absurd concept to believe in. To the Stoics, health is part of what is referred to as "preferred indifferents" (along with things such as fame and riches). Conversely, "dispreferred indifferents" I see as including poverty, death, ugliness, weakness and fragility. However, these things are still not bad.

Health is morally indifferent but holds *some* value and desire. We cannot see health as "good", as it has potential to be "bad". To clarify, "indifferent" is a specialised word which means that the relevant thing doesn't contribute in any way to genuine fulfilment or to its opposite, dissatisfaction. If we flip a coin there is a 50 per cent chance that it will land on heads; but it is perfectly possible that on flipping the coin ten times, it won't fall on heads once. Each time the coin is flipped it becomes another individual incident holding a 50 per cent chance – even with 100,000 flips. We can take control of ourselves through means of exercise and the consumption of nutritious food, but the "coin of health" always has the chance of landing on the side of trouble.

The overall purpose of physical improvement for the Stoics was similar to that taught by Socrates – acuity of the mind. "The greater the load, moreover, on the body is crushing to the spirit and renders it less active. So keep the body within bounds as much as you can and make room for the spirit." In this quotation, Seneca is telling us that overtraining is the inevitable consequence of faulty prioritisation, and it will leave little room for the spirit (such as the psychological harm of muscle dysmorphia).

Overtraining can lead to an obsession of ego. Although an addicted athlete is not a slave to a drug or a substance of any sort, he is still a slave to his own passions and desires. Arguably these passions are healthier than, say, overeating, but realistically they are just as morally bad. The Adonis Complex shows us that much of this harm is psychological and not directly visible to the spectator. Society's groupthink mentality opposes any argument against serious attachment; likewise with sex as it is defined mostly as good. From this arises a difficulty in actually vocalising any psychological struggle. The struggle of being "too fit" is difficult for most to accept or even understand, and could perhaps even cause ridicule ("fit shaming"). But of course, for a great majority this is not the problem. Still, I think it's important to recognise, as anyone can get to this point.

SYMBOLS OF MASCULINITY

Stoicism may conjure up a philosophy that is as tough and emotionless as the English word *stoic*. This definition has intertwined into the definition of masculinity itself. For an individual who is unhealthy and overweight it can become a very difficult task to make any significant progress because the thought of discussing personal issues may instigate a sense of vulnerability which men specifically have been trained to never expose.

There is an icon in our society which stands out – "beer and sports". While this is normal (and there is nothing inherently wrong with showcasing and promoting hobbies that tailor towards the natural interests of men – including my own), there's a danger in cultivating a hegemonic view over a very unhealthy practice and the entertainment of sport (a healthy practice). The harm comes when "sport" and "beer" can't exist without each other.

The act of drinking per se is symbolic of the masculine. We could argue that drinking alcohol is a risky practice, so wouldn't it make sense that more masculine people (perceived as being more inclined to take risks) will drink in excess? My answer is that I don't think alcohol has anything to do with masculinity in any natural way, just as birds don't have anything to do with coffee. The attachment came about through the homosocial glue of sports and other behaviours which are now seemingly indivisible.

Changes such as the criminalisation of drink-driving suggest that within society drinking is gradually losing the masculine aura it has always been associated with. Psychoanalytical researchers largely agree that many people considered alcoholics are simply men who are over reliant on alcohol as a crutch to compensate for subconscious feelings of male inadequacy. Of course this isn't true in every case, but it's interesting to think about. A 2004 diet-controlled intervention study from the *Alcoholism: Clinical and Experimental Research* journal looked at the effect of alcohol on testosterone, dehydroepiandrosterone sulphate (DHEAS) and oestradiol levels. Interestingly, the experiment found an increase in blood testosterone levels after a small (0.5/kg) dose of alcohol. A moderate dose (which equates to 1.5 glasses of red wine) only lowered testosterone levels by 7 per cent. Perhaps the threshold of an increase/decrease of testosterone could be a determinant of what is "masculine" or not (if we were to equate masculinity to testosterone).

A quantitative study in 1998 by the *Australian and New Zealand Journal of Public Health* showed that the older generation coming out of World War II had a frequent habit of concealing their pain. This conclusion was made through the observation of older men's concerns with their urological health. A clear tendency existed with participants concealing pain in order to uphold the image of a stronger character. Showing reaction was symbolic of weakness. A very large body of empirical evidence supports the notion that men are reluctant to seek help elsewhere (especially from health professionals). Depression, substance abuse, physical disabilities and general stress are issues that men are particularly reluctant to seek help for, in comparison to women. Experts believe this is the reason men are much more likely to actually follow through with suicidal thoughts.

Researcher Carole Pinnock tells us that respondents in the study spoke of "suffering" and "making do". The subjects described feelings of isolation, embarrassment and having pride ultimately disturb their peace of mind. This constant and agonising non-disclosure of issues in order to "take care" of pride and appear stoic provokes nothing but unnecessary suffering for a man who cannot feel it to be part of his nature to submit to help. This modern definition of stoicism is commonly misrepresentative of the ancient philosophy of Stoicism.

So why is it much more difficult for men to seek help? Is it a societal narrative of masculinity constructed in a manner which forms ideologies, beliefs and norms, and dissolves what masculinity really is? Or is it that the naturally masculine seek comfort through silence and an empty glass? Is one morally superior to the other? There will always be variability in the way each man seeks help. The way men act masculine is different. The conformity to modern emotional stoicism may provoke the feeling that to ask for help is an act of surrender and defeat through the piercing of one's self-esteem and thus, a sign of weakness. Marcus Aurelius stresses the opposite: "Don't be ashamed to need help. Like a soldier storming a wall, you have a mission to accomplish. And if you've been wounded and you need a comrade to pull you up? So what?"

The common response to anguish is: "I can overcome; all I need is time." Many feel that asking for help is morally wrong

– and this can be true, depending on what the help is for and the situation one is in. There is no absolute truth in a matter with such subjective problems. However, Marcus Aurelius makes it clear that seeking help is in fact okay. He's also very clear that there is a silent agreement that must be understood. In order to seek help, we must be sure that this cry for help is grounded in an inability to help ourselves, a last resort; *not* a form of escape. Marcus doesn't tell us that for every problem we should seek help, simply that there is no shame in doing so.

I think this quotation above subtly insinuates that finding closure introspectively is the priority. It is clear that dealing with problems through excessive alcoholic consumption or through any other means of external stimuli entails nothing morally good – it is simply an *emotive* response, which opposes the essence of true masculinity. Many may argue it is "rational" to drink when sad or angry, but the fallacy of this argument is in the emotion their opinion is likely influenced by. I also don't agree with complete abstinence being the most masculine option. Having the capacity to moderate without becoming attached is the ideal.

When an individual feels embarrassed in the act of confession there is no outwards flow of emotion and a compression-type effect occurs. Then comes sadness, melancholy, lost hope and, most visible to the external world, the habits – such as drinking – which accompany these internalisations. Seneca asserts that a habit which gives a man a sense of stability is what will eventually cause fault, as the act becomes more able to entrench itself into the mind and, as he said, "take deeper roots".

Understand that Stoicism isn't an isolating philosophy. We know through Seneca's well-articulated writing that he adamantly believes that nothing delights the mind more than "true and sweet" friendship. Seneca goes on to explain that with a close friendship every secret is safe. What *is* harmful is to decide to bond with someone whose desires are far from moderate. It is the moderate we should seek to form cooperative and symbiotic relationships with. Despite any presumptions we may hold of one's character, vices within men are contagious and will spread effortlessly. Isn't it true that some diseased bodies previously came into contact with other sick bodies? It is no different for the contagious nature of the mind, which we mustn't forget is connected to the body. Only two individuals who actively renounce those things which are within and without our control can form friendships which are meaningful and fruitful. If you don't have these individuals in your life, then comes an abundance of time alone, and with solitude other problems can arise.

THE AGE OF SOCIAL ABUNDANCE?

From Greek mythology to the Bible, loneliness has always been portrayed as an experience of the human condition. Loneliness is a strange experience; most define it as sadness caused by social isolation. Personally I don't think "sadness" does justice to the nature of loneliness. We are not better or worse, more profound or insignificant, because of loneliness. What I am certain of is that loneliness isn't the result of an event, but rather a product of our nature. Being lonely is indivisible from who we are as human beings. Loneliness is not a rating system, or part of some emotive scale. It is a response to a lack of external stimuli, and is part of the human psyche.

Technological progress in modern civilisation can be frustrating. It's also intriguing to watch as our curiosity and inclination to make objectively bad decisions brings out our true human nature – just as if we'd been given a button that says "do not press".

The internet is a very, very strange thing. Seriously, think about it. Humans ("hairless pink monkeys", to quote comedian and commentator Joe Rogan) upload their conscious thoughts onto a universal platform and watch while others immediately respond and interact to them. Have we become too curious in creating something like this? The internet began as a tool for the military; but now we share, we experience, essentially we *live* so much of our lives locked into this tool. Do we reject it, or do we find a way to live life best integrated with the online sphere?

Think for a moment about the progress we have made. I was born in 1994; merely two decades have gone by and yet the world has undeniably shifted in profound ways in that time. In the past, 500-year increments meant nothing. Are we developing too quickly? Is our curiosity our enemy?

I believe we need to rethink our lives the moment the popularity of philosophies such as Stoicism and Buddhism come to the mainstream. The purpose of such philosophies is to ground and recalibrate ourselves into our nature. Stoicism, in particular, directs a pupil in the direction of nature. What is so ironic is that we are reteaching ourselves to live naturally, using the means that created dissonance with nature in the first place. To further the absurdity, look above at the paragraph you just read and think of the technology which allowed me to conjure and express this very thought with you. Yes, I know you get it; the world today is a strange place.

We are reminded of how ever so connected we are on a daily basis – yet the disconnection is ever so clear. In an instant, one can connect to another. Whenever we feel even one squirm of uncomfortable isolation, then comes the instantaneous act of using the medium of the internet in order to *not* deal with that which will later deepen the very void attempting to be filled. The experience of being lonely – the feeling, the instant when you realise you are the definition of the word itself – I see as having potential to be comforting. Loneliness is a part of human nature; one man is no different to another in his nature and so we all experience it. So what is there to be lonely about?

When I first form a picture of the word *lonely* in my mind I imagine exclusion, I visualise a man alone, in darkness, isolated, likely apprehensive. There is lack of human touch, lack of connection, lack of oxytocin, and falling more deeply in love with the fantasy of social abundance; but today this definition is changing. Loneliness is becoming a paradox – many of us have a goal of making as many social connections as possible within the shortest period of time, and this is essentially the root of loneliness itself. This way of thinking warrants no appreciation for what patience and care bring to forming unbreakable bonds with a few worthwhile people, which will always be more fruitful and genuine than an arbitrary number, online and in person, could ever be.

The fact that we are able to make what appears to be human contact in any given situation, at any hour of the day, means we have a much less likely chance of making the same amount of *real* physical encounters. An antisocial generation has been born, for whom it is *not* normal to reach out and physically touch someone with their hands.

This outstanding growth of isolation is parallel to the exponential growth of technology, specifically the popularity of social media, and alcoholic consumption which I think appears to be the variable keeping our sociability intact. In the United States, 18.3 per cent of Americans were categorised as binge drinkers in 2012, an increase of nearly 9 per cent since 2005.

Wide empirical evidence suggests that women, who tend to be more affectionate and in need of physical touch, use the internet more – particularly spending more time on social media fostering social connections. Furthermore, what is fascinating to note is that people who frequently check Facebook on their smartphone tend to have less grey matter of the nucleus accumbens (a reward-related area of the brain) according to a 2012 study from the *Behavioural Brain Research Journal*. It should be pointed out that further studies are needed to decipher exactly what the effect of a decrease of grey matter is in relation to use of Facebook. The nucleus accumbens plays an important role in motivation and reward (i.e., incentive and positive reinforcement). It could be that the "seeking activity," as the study phrased it, through pleasure gained from fostering social connections, is parallel in some way to the mechanism of the brain's reward system, similar to alcoholic consumption. (This point is just a supposition on my part as research has not got us this far yet, although I think that the manic and stimulating nature of Facebook is actually contributing to the various factors affecting obesity's rise. This may sound strange, but you'll understand this idea by the end of the book.)

Clearly there's something to be concerned about, when studies are conclusive that these "reward systems" (such as Facebook) have such powerful effects on the brain.

According to psychologist John Cacioppo and his colleagues from the University of Chicago, extreme loneliness increases people's chances of premature mortality by 14 per cent. This number is nearly as significant as that of socio-economic status, which stands at 19 per cent. These numbers rival that of the impact of obesity. It's odd that something that we seem to take for granted and quickly disassociate from the body can affect how long we live. Isolation, worry, feeling as if nobody cares for you – these feelings result in physical impairment due to elevations in blood pressure, disturbed sleeping patterns and increased cortisol secretion in the morning. Cacioppo tells us that those suffering loneliness experience increased depression and even alteration in the expression of immune cells.

In Stoicism, loneliness isn't something that we should avoid. A man should be content with a life lived in solitude. Why? Because sometimes being alone is better than being around those who are not good for us. I suspect some of the injury to health arises from the *perception* of loneliness; the stigma, the social narrative which then lowers our status below others who are perceived to live in social abundance.

Epictetus said: "Nevertheless, a man should also be prepared to be sufficient unto himself – to dwell with himself alone, even as God dwells with Himself alone, shares His repose with none, and considers the nature of His own administration, intent upon such thoughts as are meet unto Himself. So should we also be able to converse with ourselves, to need none else beside, to sigh for no distraction, to bend our thoughts upon the Divine Administration, and how we stand related to all else; to observe how human accidents touched us of old, and how they touch us now; what things they are that still have power to hurt us, and how they may be cured or removed; to perfect what needs perfecting as Reason would direct."

In other words, it's not loneliness that is the problem – it's how you *feel* about it. We can control the relationships we have with people, so that despite a lack of social connection we can make the decision to not be lonely because of it. This doesn't mean that we should avoid social relationships as long as we perceive loneliness correctly. The point is that if a situation in your life arises where social isolation is most conducive to living according to nature, then breathe easy, knowing that you really do have control over your perception of it.

For children, human touch is magical. Touch is essential from the moment we are born and through our development during infancy. It is now accepted that touch is a precursor to the expression of ailment or good health as an adult. A 2010 review from *Infant Behavior and Development* found that premature infants who were massaged for fifteen minutes three times per day gained weight at a rate 47 per cent greater than those isolated in incubators. Touch indicates safety. Babies cannot articulate themselves and thus touch becomes the replacement for this human expression.

Outside sexual encounters, how important is physical touch to adults? Apes and monkeys, who are our close animal relatives, spend upwards of one-fifth of their day grooming and touching each other. Robin Dunbar in his book *Grooming, Gossip, and the Evolution of Language*, tells us that when apes groom and touch for such a long period of time, it's not just about hygiene. They also do this to tighten their social bonds. What is fascinating about Dunbar's argument is his claim that we developed languages to replace this sort of bonding because "social grooming" made impossible demands on our time as we advanced intellectually.

It could be said that we live in a time in which social grooming is predominately electronic. Yet there are things that cannot be expressed in words, and at that point we often go back to our primate roots and use physical touch as a means to bond and become close. (Unfortunately, for many people, alcohol is usually required for this to happen). Increasingly, our electronic-centric lives cannot fulfil this desire and it isn't a change one can simply get used to within ten years, as the need for touch is part of our DNA.

When touched, a person's production of oxytocin increases. Oxytocin is a peptide hormone, released in largest quantities during orgasm, but also through friendship and mutual communicating. It's even administered as medication during childbirth. The release of oxytocin creates calm, and allows people to trust and love – but these levels of secretion cannot be replicated through an electronic screen.

I came across an interesting documentary on VICE a couple of years ago about a new phenomenon in Japan called "cuddle cafés". In these cafés people pay money to cuddle other people. It is not a brothel. It is explicitly for the social aspect (no happy endings are included). Japan is one of the most socially isolated countries in the world with a population of more than 126 million and more than 115 million internet users, meaning Japan has 91.1 per cent "internet penetration". Japan is a country that some would say rewards introverted behaviour; a different phenomenon from the West, but something which is becoming more common and accepted in Western countries (being a couch potato is the new "cool"). South Korea is in a similar position with a comparable culture to Japan in this aspect.

What really grabbed my attention was the perspective Japanese people have on the moral acceptance of drinking. A

2014 survey conducted by the Pew Research Center for the Global Attitudes Project, asked people from forty countries for their moral beliefs on drinking alcohol. The options were: acceptance, rejection, or not relevant. Those countries that most rejected alcohol were all Muslim countries (Pakistan, followed by the Palestinian territories and Indonesia.) Japan came out on top by a significant margin on the opposite spectrum with 66 per cent saying drinking is morally acceptable, while only 6 per cent adamantly opposed it.

Many people aren't willing to completely abstain from alcohol. With this mindset comes the importance of approaching such a commonly abused substance with the right approach.

Eubulus (fourth century BC) was a comic poet from Athens. In one of his plays Dionysus says, "Three bowls do I mix for the temperate: one to health, which they empty first; the second to love and pleasure; the third to sleep. When this bowl is drunk up, wise guests go home. The fourth bowl is ours no longer, but belongs to violence; the fifth to uproar; the sixth to drunken revel; the seventh to black eyes; the eighth is the policeman's; the ninth belongs to biliousness; and the tenth to madness and the hurling of furniture."

The idea is that three bowls is the ideal quantity of wine to drink. What is important to understand is that this number is representative of *moderation* rather than a specific quantity. Moderation is a theme that recurs often in ancient Greek writings. The idea that alcohol is something which will either be misused or used appropriately is an ancient concept. What this quotation shows is that the more you drink the more harmful it will be for you.

Moderation comes from the conscious decision to stop pouring when the time is right. Eubulus explains that it is important to think before you act out of emotional compulsion. What this guideline *isn't* is a literal outline of how much you should be drinking, as a *kylikes* (drinking cup) is diluted with water and is a different size from the normal glass we use today. The appropriate quantity for you is dependent on your body weight, metabolism, tolerance and other genetic factors which predispose certain individuals to become more intoxicated than others.

Moderation comes from self-awareness in moments of decisions, which align themselves to progressive phases – Eubulus' "one to health", "the second to love" and "the tenth to madness and the hurling of furniture." – in congruence with your unique physiology. A Stoic may consume wine when relaxing and resting but does *not* get drunk. On the odd occasion, a man may endure the temporary insanity of the drunken state and experience the melancholy which follows. What is important in this scenario is to understand that a wise man does not grieve over the matter, or even regret it. Remember, time is a like a river, when something happens it will continue flowing down the stream; don't be foolish enough to swim upstream.

The Stoic school of philosophy proposes that emotions should be avoided in favour of intellect. There is nothing unmasculine in eating healthy and living a healthy lifestyle, nor is there in moderation of alcoholic consumption. Being able to moderate yourself is based on the decision to go with what is most logical for improved longevity. But moderation doesn't get in the way of living a completely abnormal life which may result in another type of harm.

Seneca says something rather thought-provoking, something the average university student ought to take note of: "It shows much more courage to remain dry and sober when the mob is drunk and vomiting; but it shows greater self-control to refuse to withdraw oneself and to do what the crowd does, but in a different way – thus neither making oneself conspicuous nor becoming one of the crowd." The idea is simply that restriction of something such as alcohol doesn't mean one must also restrict themselves from the (very fun) activities often associated with drinking, whether this is spending time with friends or visiting cool locations around the city.

THE WAR ON EGO

We experience reality through everything around us: the material objects we touch, what we buy, the environment around us. We experience this reality in relation to ourselves, through what we could call the *ego* – not in the Freudian sense; instead I define this term as an inflated sense of self-importance. The ego is the bad-tempered child-like persona that lies within. It is this childish voice that has a deep desire for recognition. Maybe you're an athlete, maybe you're rich and in poor health, maybe you're the editor helping me with this book; whoever you are, this childish voice screams "not me!" as you read this very line.

But this darker side of the psyche exists in us all. It is a part of ourselves that should be understood rather than silenced. If we understand it, we can manage it. Whether we want to accept it or not, the ego collectively runs our economy; it is the decision maker of contemporary civilisation and our world's collective consciousness. The ego is the entity that is personified through our individual decisions that we wholeheartedly believe to be our own.

Many make the erroneous assumption that there's no difference between the self and the ego. Self is further beyond the ego and is deeper and indifferent. The ego should be seen like a mirror. It's defined, not by the self, but rather by the myriad of experiences that the self watches float by. The self is where dreams come from; it's everything that's you. The self is instinct, intuitive, the spiritual manifestations that extend further beyond our materialistic nature. The self is the spectator to your life experiences, the silent observer; it is the fraction of the cosmos that we all share. The self is your inner "spark of rationality".

There is a never-ending antagonism between the self and

the ego. In every battle, in every sport and competition, there is an aggressor. There is one side which seeks to dominate, while the other defends. It is the ego that provokes the self, as only the ego has an agenda. The ego is constantly trying to make the self submit; it fights to accept the ego-driven reality we live in as honest and pure. The more you can move your perception of reality towards the self which has no judgement and no illusions, the greater your fulfilment and joy will be; and the less you will be a slave to motives of the external. The self works on energy, which is universal – indifference and rationale are its imperatives. We must make a conscious effort to fight in this war against the ego, while completely accepting that the war will never be won.

On the journey of improving your health, at some point it will become apparent to others that you are changing. This may be the changing shape of your body; but more often it's your character. I've noticed that whatever change is most visible, will receive the largest attention. In general people don't want others to change, as this distorts the fantasies we like to project onto others. We project these fantasies because categorising people is an instinctual habit. When we know the behaviour of another person we improve the predictability and thus the security of the reality we live in. Since so many of us base our actions on the perspectives of others, people rarely change.

If anyone treats you ill, speaks ill of you directly or indirectly, this is not an attack on you. This is simply a vocalisation of what they believe to be their duty. Any incorrect insult to your efforts is simply a fault. The accuser becomes the one who is hurt; he is the one unfortunate as he is deceived. Seneca asserts that in such a situation one must simply think to himself: "It seemed so to him." For instance, let's say someone were to say, "I am stronger than you, so therefore I am better than you." You may very well take this to heart. This phrase is simply illogical. "I am stronger than you, so I am better than you", is fallacious. Instead, what does make sense is saying, "I am stronger than you, therefore I can lift more weight than you." Perhaps they will never phrase it in this way, but you can interpret it through this perspective.

The journey of improving yourself through physical exercise is a great weapon to use in this war. By lifting weights, running, competing in sport and improving your health, you can choose to go in favour of the ego or the self. The ego may seek to improve your body for others, to impress potential partners and/or for validation. The self seeks to improve for the integrity of your character. You will eventually understand the difference between the ego and the self through building your body, but for some this can come too late and at a cost of self-degeneration through the use of anabolic androgens (steroids).

The ego isn't necessarily always bad – but we need to keep a balance. To be aware of the ego without falling under its sovereignty gives us power and control over our pursuits. When you are competing against others, essentially you are favouring your ego, but if the ego is inflated strategically you can then use this to compete to benefit yourself. As Stoic philosopher Chrysippus says: "He who is running a race ought to endeavour and strive to the utmost of his ability to come off victor; but it is utterly wrong for him to trip up his competitor, or to push him aside. So in life it is not unfair for one to seek for himself what may accrue to his benefit; but it is not right to take it from another."

The key is to remain disconnected from this desire elsewhere, but utilise it in the moment. When faced with your inner compulsion to compete, your victory should not derive from beating other people. This is why exercise with the self, through weightlifting, swimming and running, gives you the opportunity to experience satisfaction through overcoming your own boundaries. The result is a victory over yourself and with a win over others being secondary. The objective is to dominate, but to do so humbly.

For the ego, it doesn't matter whether attention is positive or negative; no matter what, it will still crave the attention. This attention comes as a sense of entitlement and boosted self-importance through validation. If you listen carefully while you walk the streets or sit in a cafe, most people constantly discuss topics surrounding themselves – what *I* wish to pursue in the future and what *I* have accomplished, what *I* intend to do for my benefit: *me, me, me*. The majority of what people say has no substance and, as Marcus Aurelius tells us, it is best to "be silent for the most part, or, if you speak, say only what is necessary and in a few words". I'm guilty of this myself! Everyone is, but too often silence is what says the most.

Silence seems to be interpreted by many people to be a bad thing, as it means attention is diverted away from them. Despite the attention even possibly being negative, if it is shifted away from us, the ego craves it. Silence is a state the ego will persistently manipulate us into perceiving as vulnerability. Silence is a loss of opportunity to shift ourselves back into the spotlight, to continue bringing attention towards ourselves.

Do not speak of your ambitions; let your actions speak for themselves. No matter how little you have done, words are easy to produce. You can say anything you want about yourself – it means nothing. Become comfortable with silence; let others take the attention and let your ego dissolve into its rightful place while you *actually* accomplish and follow through with your intentions.

Think of silence as an exercise in self-discipline, which Stoics call *askesis*. Now, silence isn't necessarily a virtue in itself – we are social creatures and this will never change. But simply be aware of when it is required to speak and do so with purpose. Zeno tells us that we were born with two ears and one mouth, yet most choose to speak more than they listen. Ask yourself whether your words are somehow contributing or whether they are taking away from your own self-worth.

"It is impossible for a man to learn what he thinks he already knows," Epictetus says. And of course there is the famous

Socratic paradox: "I know that I know nothing." We could call this the antonym of the ego. If you claim to have "perfect wisdom" you lose your ability to learn and to be a student of life. The ego protects us from learning new information as we may begin to see ourselves as all-knowing. If you think you already know everything there is to know, it becomes impossible to take in new information. The moment you humble yourself and can admit that you don't know something, this is when the learning process begins; this is when your mind is able to fully open and take in the world around it with clarity, free from bias and your own arrogance. It's only when we become comfortable with ignorance that we give ourselves the opportunity to rid ourselves of it. To learn more about your body, your health, how to take care of it, to excel, and accept that there's going to be someone that knows more about it than you. This should cultivate excitement; never resentment.

Books today are cheaper than ever, courses inexpensive too (some even free and yet still extremely valuable). There is no excuse to remain uneducated. Today there exists a myriad of historical and scientific knowledge accessible at the click of a button. Perhaps it is this lack of effort which blocks our ability to open that first page. Our ego interferes with taking this often free commodity as we fear feedback through our very own internalisations. Fear is vastly pronounced when these sources may bring out the flaws we frequently hide away. We fear disapproval and we remain hostile to feedback. Now you may question what on earth this has to do with the "Stoic body". This has everything to do with it.

The proverb "when the student is ready, the teacher will appear", is a relevant conclusion to this point. There are brilliant individuals, far more intelligent than you or I, who spent years of their life, hundreds upon hundreds of hours researching, learning and understanding our world, condensing their most profound insights into a paperback book. In these books they show their best side, their highest self and their greatest thoughts, with one goal – to spread all that they know in their particular field for the price of a few cappuccinos. Spend time educating yourself in the field you wish to improve. It is not often you find a financially ruined individual who constantly reads on economics, finance and business; and likewise it is uncommon to find an obese person well educated in nutrition and exercise.

PART TWO:
THE STOIC PALATE

"Since these and other mistakes are connected with food, the person who wishes to be self-controlled must free himself of all of them and be subject to none."

– Musonius Rufus

THE EVOLUTION OF OBESITY

n 2014, over 1.9 billion adults (those aged 18 years and over) were overweight, and over 600 million of these overweight individuals were classified as being obese. Worldwide, obesity has more than doubled since 1980. These figures were calculated using the Body Mass Index (BMI). The BMI uses the following formula:

$$\frac{(\text{Weight in pounds [lbs]} \times 703)}{(\text{Height in inches} \times \text{height in inches})}$$

The World Health Organisation (WHO) defines 18.5-24.9 on the BMI as normal; 25-29 is overweight and anything greater than 30 is categorised as obese. This formula isn't completely accurate as it doesn't distinguish between a person's fat and muscle. A very muscular individual could be classed as overweight according to the BMI, for example. However, what the BMI does is provides us with the best representation of overall demographic trends on a population-wide scale.

Just as we are looking into the past for wisdom from the Stoics, we should also look into our evolutionary past to understand the fundamental reasons why we are in this situation in the first place. The *drifty gene hypothesis* was proposed in 2007 by John Speakman, a British biologist, in critique of the *thrifty gene hypothesis*, postulated by James V Neel in 1962. Speakman argues that because hominids thousands of years ago had their selection pressure revoked from them, this essentially formed the basis for our contemporary obesity epidemic. Advances in both intellect and technology have seen humans exist well outside of their intended nature. The issue of obesity comes partially from our instinctual drive for survival, with sugar being our most preferred source of energy.

Harvard evolutionary biologist Daniel Lieberman, author of *The Story of the Human Body: Evolution, Health, and Disease*, tells us that sugar is a "deep, deep ancient craving". He claims we are programmed in a way that causes us to gain weight as it is a natural and "positive" adaptation for improving the chances of survival.

Sugar is a vague term. For example, sucrose (table sugar) consists of one molecule of glucose and another of fructose. Fruits are generally a mixture of glucose and fructose, but this varies depending on the fruit.

Glucose is what dominates the blood (you've probably heard of "blood glucose" in reference to diabetics). Chimpanzees, who are considered one of our closest relatives in the animal kingdom, live on insects and leaves, but predominately fruit.

I recently interviewed three neuroscientists/medical doctors. The first said humans are herbivores, the second said we're carnivores and the third said we're omnivores, ha! I personally believe we are omnivorous. Regardless of what you believe it's clear sugar tastes good to us because of a deep desire we have for it.

According to Speakman, since we are out of the equation of natural selection, our genes (which dictate energy storage), have "drifted" through our genetic lineage. Increasingly research is pointing towards the addictive-like behaviour in individuals being more about the food palate reward, rather than the sugar itself; but the relevant point is that we have reached a point in our society where the naturally occurring scarcity of commodities such as sugar is no longer applicable. Society has adapted far quicker than our genes ever could and survival has now become an expectation.

Gaius Musonius Rufus (AD 25–95) was a Roman Stoic who taught during the reign of Nero. Musonius tells us that "the pleasure connected with food is undoubtedly the most difficult of all pleasures to combat". He was known to speak about the topic of food frequently, having written an entire two-part discourse dedicated to the subject of food. What we can interpret from his dialogue is that as an activity we partake in every single day, food naturally becomes a frequent test of *sophrosyne* (soundness of the mind, leading to purity, self-control and prudence). Musonius Rufus tells us: "Indeed the throat was designed to be a passage of food, not an organ of pleasure, and the stomach was made for the same purpose as the root was created in plants. For just as the root nourishes the plant by taking food from without, so the stomach nourishes the plant by taking food and drink which are taken into it."

In his lectures Musonius Rufus speaks of the importance of having a diet which is based on plant-based sources. He advocated limiting the consumption of meat, reasoning that meat "darkens the soul." To Musonius, meat is a heavy food and places too much difficulty on our digestive system and slows down our ability to think clearly and rationally. I am not one to advocate one specific type of diet as you will find later in this chapter; but a lot of evidence today points towards the overconsumption of meat, especially processed red meat (which has been categorised as a carcinogen), clearly doing more harm than good.

The term *wholefoods* describes natural, unprocessed foods with few ingredients which can be counted on one hand. "Can I pick this off a tree?" or, "Can I kill this in a forest?" These are questions you should be asking yourself, and if the answer is yes, then you have a wholefood. This isn't to suggest that anything manufactured in an unnatural manner in the slightest way should be forbidden; rather, aiming to consume mostly wholefoods should act as your foundation. Because let's be honest, nearly every food today can fit under the definition of processed. Living this way you can save a lot of time through the tedious nature of being able to "fit all your calories in".

Wholefoods help you to feel full. A good example is beans. Beans have a decent proportion of protein and fibre and satiate your stomach, as they literally expand inside you. By contrast, many processed foods have little nutritional value and are often referred to as "empty" calories. Although not completely useless per se, you should always strive not to "see what I can get away with" but to eat food which is healthy. Doctor and author Mark Hyman, in his book *The UltraMind Solution*, shows us that much of our depressions, anxieties and even ADHD are connected to what we put into our bodies. There are far too many benefits lost when disregarding the importance of what the food actually is comprised of.

During World War I troops were fed by canned and preserved food. Post-WWI, we experienced the revolution of convenience as we progressed into the roaring twenties. Michael Pollan, author of *The Omnivore's Dilemma*, says: "So we find ourselves as a species almost back to where we started: anxious omnivores struggling once again to figure out what it is wise to eat." We are told by nutritionists and trainers to look at the labels on our food, and rightly so. On a daily basis people are manipulated by carefully crafted and packaged marketing, emphasising words like "natural" in bright colours on the front of charming and intoxicating packaging (while some variation of sugar is in fine print somewhere obscure). "One hundred per cent natural" means that the product originated from a natural source, but in many cases this does not exclude artificial additives later in processing.

This constant negotiation we have between ourselves and the choices we are making forges an unhealthy relationship with food. We forget that we are *supposed* to make decisions through our sight, smell and instinct. It's a struggle for me to tell people to count their calories; in the short term yes, but please don't let this internal negotiation become your way of getting by. It is useful to do every few weeks, especially when you are new, in order to recalibrate your alignment with your dietary demands. If counting calories is something you know will help you stay consistent, then do it. Plug "IIFYM calorie calculator" into Google. It's self-explanatory and as reliable as they get. It will ask for your body fat percentage. Simply google different percentages and find someone with a similar body for a rough estimate.

THE LUCK OF THE FRENCH

As I write these very words I am sitting in a cafe in Paris. I've been in the French capital for less than forty-eight hours; I have seen thousands of people within the last day, none of whom – and I mean zero – were even remotely obese. I am witnessing what is known as the *French paradox*. This paradox is the riddle of the French people's low rates of coronary heart disease (CHD) despite high consumption of foods rich in saturated fats. The term itself was coined in the newsletter of *International Organisation of Vine and Wine* in 1986. Frank Cooper in the book *Cholesterol and the French Paradox* argues that this epidemiological phenomenon is based on French people's consumption of natural saturated fats, such as butter, which to many is symbolic of weight *gain*.

It is no secret that the French enjoy their wine. Red wine contains polyphenols. The antioxidant components of red wine, such as resveratrol, proanthocyanidins and quercetin are protective against oxidation and inflammation which is associated with atherosclerotic lesions. This is one important reason why red wine is advantageous over spirits, beer and even white wine, and perhaps explains the lower cardiovascular disease rates in France.

In his book *The Fat Fallacy: the French Diet Secrets to Permanent Weight Loss*, written in 2003, Will Clower makes the argument that the French paradox can be narrowed down to several points. Overall the French eat less sugar, more "good" fats than "bad" and don't have the same access as much of the Western world to the ridiculous variety of takeaway food items at cheap prices. The French eat slower, with smaller portions. The courses of French meals are divided in a way that allows the body to digest previous consumed food before more food is added. Being "full" to the French is not the purpose. Furthermore, the French eat fewer snacks between meals (eating only when necessary), take longer breaks between meals and spend far longer in actually preparing a meal from home. I think that the food culture in France simply embraces the quality of food over quantity.

The French defend the quality of their food. The Appellation d'Origine Contrôlée (AOC) is a controlled designation of origin, which applies to a variety of foods such as red wine, butter and seafood. This regulation is in place to control the quality of products.

I was travelling in Thailand with a friend of mine who enjoys eating quickly and has an abnormal appetite. We were on a hike in northern Thailand, and stayed briefly on a passion fruit farm. By coincidence we were housed with a group of French tourists. It was interesting for me to observe the difference between my friend – an example of what *not* to do for the obese – and the French people, who ate only one piece of toast for breakfast. My friend, who was baffled at the absurdity of their breakfast choices, asked, "Aren't you still hungry?" The French travellers were baffled at both how fast and how much my friend could eat. (I must say, this interaction was hilarious to watch.)

Italians have an appreciation for food similar to that of the French. A study from Leicester University found that although life expectancy is similar across Europe, Italians live healthier for longer. The study came to the conclusion that men from Italy will live healthier for ten years longer than British men, while Italian women live healthier for fourteen more years than British women. The researchers believed there were various reasons for this; but emphasised that Italians spend more time preparing and enjoying their food, instead of the average of just fifteen minutes of food preparation in Britain.

FAT, DAIRY AND CHOLESTEROL

In 2012, research from the *European Journal of Nutrition* examined whether high-fat dairy diets had any correlation to obesity, cardiovascular disease and various other metabolic disorders. The conclusion was that high-fat dairy did not increase risk of metabolic disease and actually lowered the risk of obesity. During follow-ups of nearly 350,000 subjects of research, a meta-analysis in 2010 from the American Society for Nutrition concluded that there is no significant evidence that dietary saturated fat is correlated with an increased risk of CHD or CVD.

Butter from grass-fed cows is rich in vitamin K2. A deficiency of vitamin K2 increases the risk for cardiovascular disease, cancer and osteoporosis. Butter is also rich in conjugated linoleic acid (CLA), often marketed as a fat-loss supplement. It has been shown to have anti-cancer properties, and, in some studies, has lowered body fat, although there are some studies which say there is a neutral effect. Certainly none of the studies show clear negatives. Butter tastes good because fat in a meal will help us absorb and taste other potentially beneficial nutrients. However, too much saturated fat can most certainly be bad.

After getting deep into the research it appears that butter is not as healthy as coconut oil or extra-virgin olive oil if we're referring to LDL cholesterol (known as "bad cholesterol") but in moderate quantities it seems that high-fat dairy products such as butter have been demonised. HDL and LDL, which you've likely heard of, aren't actually different variations of cholesterol; these are simply proteins which carry cholesterol and triglycerides around the body.

We are often told that consuming saturated fat and cholesterol will increase your chances of having a heart attack. For years the American Medical Association backed this ideology and rejecting it seemed nonsensical. For so long the dogmatic idea existed that eating fat was parallel to its expression physiologically. I saw this with my father while I was growing up. He took medicine for his high cholesterol and would never – and I mean never – eat the yolk of an egg in fear of, well, dying. But cholesterol is being revealed as a beneficial nutrient. A deficiency of cholesterol leads to some extremely negative side effects. Now I'm not saying we should strive to increase it, but be aware that there is widespread paranoia about the consumption of cholesterol. Take the egg yolk that my father was so afraid of. It contains brain-building fats (lecithin and phospholipids) and vitamins A and D, as well as other essentially fatty acids in free-range selections.

Breast milk has large amounts of cholesterol – what does this say about nature's intentions? Surely if it's a dietary source of cancer and death, nature would have more sympathy with its first caloric commodity for infants.

It's true that there is a lot of controversy over the role of cholesterol in health. However, I have established certain things from doing extensive research on the subject, but I would be a fool to say this is the definitive answer. Nutrition is always changing and we really do need clinical trials to make definitive claims. This is simply the conclusion i've come to from interviewing experts and looking through the literature. I suggest you do your own research too. It seems that inflammation is what causes atherosclerosis; cholesterol helps to heal lesions – and is then observed as being in high concentrations when one has heart disease. Cholesterol is at the crime scene but it isn't the criminal! I won't begin to go down this rabbit hole; instead I'll point you into the direction of some leading experts from both opposing sides of the argument so you can decide what is most reasonable for you a video I recommend is by Dr Rhonda Patrick. Just search for "the cause of heart disease, Dr. Rhonda Patrick" on YouTube and you'll find it.

A common argument against dairy is that humans are the only animals which drink the milk of other animals. True. But this in itself doesn't mean it's unhealthy. Dairy consumption and bone health is something nutritional science has actually established, and the fact that osteoporosis is scarce in countries with low dairy consumption doesn't mean this isn't true – this is only a correlation.

However, 75 per cent of the world's population is estimated to be lactose intolerant (to varying degrees). Generally those of northern European descent tolerate dairy well and those of Asian descent are intolerant.

A 2016 meta-analysis from the *Food and Nutrition Research* journal explored the totality of scientific evidence over the last few decades, looking at randomised controlled trials as well as observational studies. The meta-analysis looked at the risk for various diseases, including type 2 diabetes, cardiovascular disease, osteoporosis, cancer and even all-cause mortality – all the diseases which are closely related to dietary intake. To paraphrase their conclusion: dairy and milk products were foods which contributed to daily dietary requirements and actually protect against most prevalent chronic diseases, and few adverse effects were reported.

However, dairy is not all good despite this finding, and we'll get to this in a second. First of all, if you're going to eat dairy then grass-fed is the ideal option. Grass-fed dairy is higher in vitamin K2, which helps regulate the calcium in dairy, which is important for heart and bone health. Additionally the higher concentrations of omega-3 and CLA are potentially beneficial.

In my opinion, the question of whether dairy is healthy comes down to your tolerance to it. But it's also about the quantity. Too much dairy will most likely wreak havoc on the diversity of your gut microbiome if it's not natural probiotic yogurt or organic whole milk. If you have an intolerance to gluten it's likely you're also intolerant to dairy, as milk proteins cross-react with gluten. The more compromised your gut or intestinal permeability is, the more likely your immune system is going to have trouble with butyrophilin and alpha/beta-casein (which can be allergenic). Too much dairy for many will cause discomfort and stomach aches. Dairy has nutrients which can be consumed elsewhere without these unwanted effects.

If we're specifically talking about milk then it's important to establish that all milk is *not* created equal. Natural, whole milk contains the enzyme needed to digest lactose, so it's the processing of milk which provokes lactose intolerance, not the milk itself. But we must remember that it's not wise to drink raw milk as the risk of bacterial contamination is generally regarded as too high to be advocated as being safe, when compared to something like the risk of salmonella contamination in eggs.

Dairy increases insulin and IGF-1 (insulin-like growth factor 1). Many associate this increase with the anecdotes of people having increased acne after consuming dairy. However, insulin and IGF-1 aren't always bad. For example, muscle growth is aided by insulin.

Are you more confused than ever, now? The best approach for eating dairy – and any food product which you're unsure of

– is to simply go through the process of elimination. Try and eliminate dairy for twenty to thirty days. If you feel better, then continue as you are. If you feel no different, then continue as you were. It's different for everyone.

Foods to Always Avoid

Each food product below has a rating next to it. A rating of 10 means you should *never* consume it; 1 means you should eat an abundance of it.

1. High Fructose Corn Syrup (HFCS)

Rating: 8/10

High fructose corn syrup is almost the same as plain sugar. It's found in soft drinks and other processed foods. Try to avoid this. The high concentrations of fructose are particularly bad for the health of your liver.

2. Seed and Vegetable Oils

Rating: 7/10

Soybean, cottonseed and sunflower are "healthy" oils which should be avoided like the plague. They tend to cause inflammation. These polyunsaturated fats are high in omega-6 which is something we have far too much of. The average Western diet contains a ratio of 16:1 omega-6 to omega-3, when the previous ratio was 1:1. Too much omega-6 causes inflammation and inflammation is one of the largest precursors to many diseases.

Instead opt for fatty fish, egg yolks, flaxseed, nuts such as walnuts which are particularly high in omega-3. Fats such as coconut oil, grass-fed butter and extra-virgin olive oil can be great for cooking, but try your best to get more omega-3 in your diet.

3. ARTIFICIAL SWEETENERS.

Rating: 6-7/10

Artificial sweeteners are tricky as there are various types, and many don't have any effects on your weight directly. However, there is a significant portion of evidence suggesting they may not do any good for the diversity of your gut. As you may know, 90 per cent of your serotonin is produced in your gut, 70 per cent of your immune system is in the gut, your gut even has neurons like the brain and is often referred to as the second brain. The lesson here is that the gut is intimately connected with the brain and so we should take care of the gut to take of the brain. In terms of fat loss and artificial sweeteners, I have mixed opinions on this. But as always it's probably best to stay away from artificial foods. It's better to be safe than sorry.

4. PROCESSED MEATS

Rating: 9.5/10

The World Health Organisation (WHO) has categorised processed meats as a 1A carcinogen which means they cause cancer. Red meat, according to the WHO is correlated to cancer, but not causative. Avoid processed sausages, salami, bacon where possible. Corned beef and hot dogs are other examples of processed meats. What's also important is the temperature at which you cook meat or any food for that matter. Burning food provokes carcinogenic compounds to be created.

5. TRANS FATS

Rating: 10/10

Trans fats are unsaturated fats with a very specific chemical structure. Many processed foods have these trans fats and you should avoid these completely. Not even a little bit is acceptable – trans fats are horrible for your health.

Meat and dairy, especially grass-fed variations often have small amounts of trans fat. However, these are conjugated linoleic acid or CLA which we previously established is in fact not harmful to humans. Margarine is a common source of trans fats, so instead of using margarine cook with butter.

NUTRITIONAL WARS

Smell and taste are inseparable. For Stoics, smell is one of the eight parts of the human soul. According to Dr Alan Hirsch of the Smell and Taste Research Foundation, 90 per cent of our taste is smell (think about eating when you have the flu, or try holding your nose while you eat a croissant). Smell activates deep, old parts of our brains; it is no coincidence that so many faith and religious trances are induced through the emotive scents of incense, candles and herbs. Smell acts before we think. Smell ambushes us; it conjures memories, thoughts and emotions, and heightens other senses.

Scientists believe that as humans became bipedal and moved away from sources of smells, the strength of our sense of smell came to heavily influence our behaviour. Researcher Dr Lorenzo Stafford and his team from the University of Portsmouth found that people in their sample group who were overweight had a heightened sense of smell compared to leaner people. What was fascinating about this study was the discovery that this heightened sense was exacerbated post-meal. This suggests that for the people with a propensity to gain weight, the heightened sense of smell which proceeds this feeding plays an active role in kick-starting a chain-like effect of more eating, more heightened smell and again more eating, hence an increased risk for obesity. This explains the paradoxical experience where you feel more hungry after you eat than you felt before taking your first bite.

Humans taste four flavours: bitter, sweet, sour and salty. When you're eating a food, simply describe it. Don't attach to an emotion alignment to the food; don't associate the smell with an arousal. For instance: "This cake tastes sweet" or "This food is rather salty", instead of, "This cake is soooo delicious, I can't believe how good it tastes!!!" Does the food make you feel better? Or is it giving you an experience that reflects one of the eight parts of your soul?

Musonius warns us that temptations of gluttony are before us every day. If you show no self-control over food, you risk not only your health, but your ability to control yourself in other areas. Although there are many pleasures which persuade human beings to do wrong and compel them to act against their own objective interests, the pleasure connected with food is undoubtedly one of the most difficult to resist.

As Musonius Rufus says: "That God who made man provided him food and drink for the sake of preserving his life and not for giving him pleasure, one can see very well from this: when food is performing its real function, it does not produce pleasure for man, that is in the process of digestion and assimilation."

This isn't to say that lasagne isn't pleasurable; the point is that the pleasure of food is not its true purpose. The true purpose is for digestion, energy, living and essentially surviving. When making dietary decisions, think about the implications of your choice on the true purpose of nourishment, instead of its immediate pleasure.

Try to eat lower on the food chain. This means the food will be closer to its original state, and fewer chemicals will be present in the food. Also, eat according to the seasons; eating mango during an Icelandic winter doesn't seem natural to me.

Too many people with ambitions to improve their health spend far too much time on things that provide no tangible results. As a trainer, common questions I receive are as follows: "What protein powders should I use?" or "Does X supplement work for Z results in Y amount of time?" Unless you are researching these matters purely out of curiosity or you have completely mastered consistency in the hierarchy of needs (calories → macronutrients → micronutrients → meal timing → supplements) – which is unlikely – then you have no business wasting time on such frivolous matters.

Understand that the "perfect" diet *does not* exist. For every credible study that proves one diet is better than the other, another "groundbreaking" study shows that another is indeed the best. Through the countless diet books, commercials and so-called secrets, maybe, just maybe, we are missing the point. There's a constant nutritional war between groups of people; not only based on the evidence of what is best for health, but on the ethical implications of killing animals and the environmental/agricultural effects of harvesting food. So the question is, how can you declutter the countless number of diets and find what truly works best for you? Can such a discovery even be made?

The Myth of the "Perfect Diet"

Diet simply comes down to your individual circumstances. Some people will be better off with a strict diet (for their mental cognition and peace of mind) with very occasional days off for a psychological booster. Some will adhere better to a more consistent programme if they allow themselves generous flexibility. What you should consider is how food affects you mentally. Is unhealthy food in the appropriate ratios getting you to your weight-loss goals? Great! However, ask yourself: "Is this food making me feel fatigued and lethargic?" Perhaps then it's not the most sophisticated plan for self-sustaining progress. We know on the basis of rudimentary physics that for most people (excluding those who have hormone diseases) the output/input determines fat loss/gain. We cannot sit down with a group of people and say, "For *all of you* a completely flexible diet is the best option and paleo is not!" You must try both! To attempt to determine which eating plan is best for you before trying any is setting yourself up for failure. Sure, you can make an educated guess, but you cannot guarantee a certain consequence.

If you are attempting different diets with an overlying goal of improving yourself, then that's all that is important. There is no theory that applies to everyone, as much as we might want it to. You must make it a lifestyle rather than a "four-week trans-formation". This is no different for the food you eat. Make it a lifetime journey to find what works best for you, rather than looking for a transformative quick-fix diet.

UNDERSTANDING CARBOHYDRATES AND PROTEIN

Many people have the misconception that there's something magical about a low-carbohydrate diet which somehow supersedes the laws of thermodynamics. Yes, for many people (including me), low-carb diets will be ideal. Despite how beneficial low-carbohydrate diets are perceived to be, the reason they are effective is that they provide more ideal circumstances for a caloric deficit to occur.

Think about it – when your carbohydrates are lower, your protein and fat are going to have to increase in order to compensate for the loss of calories (an example being the ketogenic diet). When you increase both of these macro-nutrients your lean body mass (LBM) retention is going to increase because of increased protein. With an increase of LBM retention comes a greater ability to maintain your basal metabolic rate (BMR). A stable BMR means a greater thermic effect of food (TEF). This thermic effect is simply the energy burned through heat which is produced from brown adipose (fat) tissue through digestive processes. If you have more fats and fewer carbohydrates in your diet, the body will slow gastric emptying. When gastric emptying is slowed your blood glucose will be more controlled (the benefit of low-carbohydrate diets). This control over glucose levels will allow you to reduce your cravings and increase satiety, but also provide stable energy throughout the day and thus a lessening of fatigue and lethargy.

Increased energy will lead to higher levels of physical activity, leading to greater energy expenditure.

You can also take into account the initial weight drop from low-carbohydrate diets within the first few days or week. Even though there's little to no change in fat loss, this drop of weight will give one the impression that a diet is working. This impression can lead to a greater adherence to a low-carbohydrate diet. Many carbohydrate-based foods are processed and dense in calories, and they rank high on the Glycaemic Index. For most, dropping carbohydrates includes these products and this will create a significant change in net calories consumed.

As you can see, low-carbohydrate diets don't work just because of insulin levels. There really is nothing special about low-carbohydrate diets. It simply comes down to the fact that lowering your carbohydrate intake affects so many other variables which creates a lifestyle more conducive (for the majority of people) to a lower overall caloric input. This is seen through higher energy expenditure, higher adherence to the diet and/or a lower caloric intake.

Contrary to common belief, there's actually no difference between sugars and complex carbohydrates – they are nutritionally identical. The difference is how quickly each is absorbed into your bloodstream.

The size of a sugar spike is dependent on two main variables: the type of food you eat and how much of it you eat. Each food receives a score out of 100 on the Glycaemic Index (GI). A low score indicates an insignificant rise in blood glucose (this is the preferred option). There's also a measurement called the Glycaemic Load (GL). The GL estimates how much a particular food will raise blood glucose levels post-ingestion.

GL and GI are important as they predict the risk of diabetes, heart disease and some cancers. As an approximate rule of thumb, anything over 50 on the GI or GL is bad, and the lower the numbers the better. When I say "bad", I am overgeneralising. I recommend you use your judgement on how natural and whole a product is. For example, some sources cite mango, pineapple and watermelon all being within a range of 56-72, yet ice cream, at 61, is lower than watermelon. Does this mean you should choose ice cream over watermelon? Of course not.

The reason why we should potentially avoid carbohydrate-rich foods and drinks is that more insulin is required to appropriately deal with the surge of glucose in the blood. Type 2 diabetes (diabetes mellitus type 2), which anyone can develop, is caused by excessive carbohydrate intake to the point where your insulin stops responding to the ridiculous amounts secreted in the body. In this situation you will find yourself joining the 392 million people worldwide (as of 2015), with type 2 diabetes, compared to around 30 million in 1985. According to the Global Burden of Disease study, type 2 diabetes makes up about 90 per cent of diabetes cases. The other 10 per cent is diabetes mellitus type 1, which is hereditary.

Dr Donald Layman, a professor of nutrition at the University of Illinois, tells us that there are benefits in eating above the recommended 56 g of protein per day. This is because protein assists muscle repair, provides satiety and prevents obesity, diabetes and heart disease (up to a certain point). Dr Mark Tarnopolsky from McMaster University tells us that athletes will thrive on 0.77 g per pound of body weight. For a 160 lb (72.5 kg) man that's 123.2 g of protein. If you are vegan or vegetarian it's possible to have an adequate protein intake; but according to Dr Tarnopolsky you need to consume 20-25 per cent more plant-based protein to compensate for what the body can actively utilise (147.84 g for the latter example). A high protein diet is generally considered one which is equal or greater than 25 per cent of total caloric intake, or 1.2–1.6 g per kilo (according to a randomised controlled study by the Journal of the American Medical Association in 2012). Often more than this can be beneficial for athletes, but there's a certain point where it becomes obsolete. A 2006 study from the Journal of the International Society of Sports Nutrition found no difference between 0.77g per pound of bodyweight versus anything over 0.91 pounds per body weight in strength, body composition or even hormones in strength athletes over three months. According to a randomised controlled trial by the Federation of American Societies for Experimental Biology in 2013, 2.4 g per kilo did not preserve lean body mass at double the recommended daily dose of 0.8 g per kilo, so 1.6 g per kilo.

The general consensus is that more protein isn't necessarily better. Despite protein raising your metabolic rate and changing some key hormones for appetite, too much is going to cause problems and even elevate the risk for some cancers. However, it may be important to increase protein intake in a caloric deficit to spare muscle loss.

Optimal protein intake actually decreases with your training age. Your body over time becomes efficient at preventing protein catabolism (breakdown) from working out and therefore less protein is needed for a smaller quantity of muscle tissue being produced post-training.

The more you exercise, the more important protein intake becomes (to a point) for adequate recovery and muscle retention. This is especially so for intense exercise.

It's important to know that protein is not made the same; there is "good" protein and "bad" protein. If you eat meat (as I do) then "good" protein would be white fish, preferably steamed, as it is low in saturated fats and rich in minerals. Fresh tuna, moderate amounts of grass-fed beef, salmon, tofu, nuts, pulses and legumes in your diet are all preferable over large quantities of red/processed meat. Even though nuts are high in calories they have the benefit of being incredibly satiating. Nuts are underrated as a source of protein. Soybeans are the best bean as it is the only one with a complete protein.

For hundreds of years people have lived as vegetarians or vegans. This was mostly based on ethics from religious and philosophical ideologies, with its roots in the ancient civilisations of Greece and India. This way of eating has almost become a philosophy in its own right today. When I was first introduced to Stoicism I began with the basics. I adopted the fundamental exercises and principles of the philosophy into my life such as negative visualisations. But when it comes to diet, Stoicism has no *nomos* (law or custom) to which I could turn to for guidance. Musonius made it very clear that we have the freedom to reject his judgement based on our own rationale.

THE MORAL HIGH GROUND

A lot of evidence to date seems to suggest that vegetarians have lower mortality rates compared to non-vegetarians. The issue with this claim is that much of the data for is population based, and can ignore other factors which may skew the results. A 2017 study from the *Preventative Medicine* journal evaluated the association between predominant categories of vegetarian diets (complete, semi- and pesco-vegetarian) and compared all-cause mortality in a population-based Australian cohort of 243,096 participants, at an average age of 62.3 years. By the 6.1 year follow-up there were 16.836 deaths and no significant difference in all-cause mortality was found for vegetarians versus non-vegetarians (including pesco- or semi-vegetarians).

So what does Stoicism teach about eating meat?

Seneca says: "I was imbued with this [vegetarian] teaching, and began to abstain from animal food; at the end of a year the habit was as pleasant as it was easy. I was beginning to feel that my mind was more active."

Seneca was a strict vegetarian until his father warned him of the social harm of being an eccentric. The Stoic philosophers who abstained from meat reasoned that we didn't truly need meat to sustain ourselves. Factually, this is true and one could argue that yes, we do have the freedom to make our own choices, but because meat (especially red meat) is more of a pleasure rather than simply being of high nutritional value, it then becomes unjust to proclaim being an ethical man and still eat meat through abundance of choice. The problem is that we can then carry this argument to anything that is pleasurable. I believe there is no need for such a restrictive and homologous ideology.

The reasons for abstaining from eating meat and animal products are many and varied. Most fall into two categories: the deontological (eating animal products is morally wrong) or the consequentialist (abstaining lessens the suffering of a fellow creature). I think the consequentialist stance is more applicable to Stoicism in certain ways. Prohibition is deontological and Stoicism is simply not based on this framework. Stoicism is based on virtue ethics.

The word *deontological* comes from the Greek *deon*, meaning one's obligation or duty. Common examples of deontological ethics are the prohibition of pork for Muslims under Islamic law; in Hinduism, beef is prohibited; another example (according to Lucian of Samosata) was that swine was prohibited in ancient Syria.

Stoic doctrine is not law. It is virtue; and virtue doesn't tell you to "not eat pork". Rather, as seen in the *Enchiridion*, we learn that we must "talk about how persons ought to eat, but eat as you ought". You make your dietary decisions on your ability to control yourself, choosing what is suitable to the appetite. Seneca says, "I do not bind myself to some particular one of the Stoic masters. I too have a right to form an opinion." Epictetus was once asked how he chose to eat, and he replied that he was "just, cheerful, equable, temperate, and orderly". Epictetus is saying that what you consume is a reflection of the virtues you hold for life.

Think about this example. Who is morally superior? Someone who eats 99 per cent plant-based soybean burgers (which require importation) or someone who eats 99 per cent whole plant-based foods and 1 per cent meat? Would the latter be the morally inferior decision to make just because the title of "vegan" isn't applicable? In fact, it's reasonable to argue that the negative consequences for the environment are likely to be more severe in the first choice. We all act to the extent at which we are comfortable restricting pleasure; this is why there is a sage ideal or perfect wisdom, one we contrast ourselves to by varying degrees based on our own affiliations, circumstances and life experiences. This is essentially why the sage is unattainable.

I agree that eating meat can be seen as a pleasure for wealthy people if a vegan diet is wholesome and taken seriously. The Stoics recognise that pleasures are unnecessary (in this case, meat) but they are still desirable (health is preferred indifferent); and so again, does that mean one should never eat a certain vegan food which isn't necessary, is pleasurable, but is damaging to the environment? How far do we take this argument? I don't believe we can take something like dietary decisions to such a deontological and absolute extreme for all. It's impossible to quantify morality in this sense in a pragmatic way.

Despite all this, I want to make something clear. Please do not believe those who tell you a vegan diet is deficient in nutrients and that veganism is therefore unhealthy. The position of the American Dietetic Association is clear: well-planned vegan and vegetarian diets are appropriate for everyone "during all stages of the life cycle, including pregnancy, lactation, infancy, childhood, and adolescence, and for athletes". More time, care and emphasis is simply needed for the provision of certain nutrients and means of preparation.

There are good reasons for reducing the consumption of meat. Processed red meat has been labelled as a potential carcinogen. Grain-fed cattle in the US have oestrogenic hormones, and other markers for ailments such as antibiotics, as well as being raised in unsanitary conditions. This doesn't mean we can *never* experience the pleasure of eating these meats. They may be unnecessary, but they can still be eaten as an occasional treat.

Grass-fed beef is quite different. It is high in vitamin E, B vitamins, conjugated linoleic acids and omega-3 fatty acids.

One health concern for Western people is the disportioncate ratio of omega-3 to omega-6, which grass-fed beef would help ameliorate. A model study called "What's Your Beef?" postulated the idea that it's possible that small farms may be carbon neutral or positive if they are regulated with a decline in meat consumption. Whether this is pragmatic for the entire world, I don't know, but it's interesting nonetheless.

We know on a psychological level that people have a greater proclivity to make changes in their life when something affects them or their immediate family directly. The average person isn't selfless enough to change habits because of an abstract term like "good for the environment. Health benefits seem to be a more rational and immediate reason.

I do think that some effort into reducing meat consumption can be argued for in the consideration of agricultural and ecological implications which does affect humanity – but I don't believe this provides enough reason for complete abstinence. We are destroying the planet and potentially our health, so choosing to eat only organic or grass-fed meat is an intelligent decision you may consider. I think most people *should* reduce their meat consumption, but telling people they're "bad" for eating meat at all is not doing your cause any favours – and it simply does not make sense. Activists could be more reasonable and say, "Hey, here are the benefits of reducing meat in your diet."

If food trends continue at their current rate then the global aim for total greenhouse gas (GHG) emissions will be surpassed by 2050. This is particularly concerning. Meat production and distribution results in excess disbursements of fuel, water, fertiliser and pesticides, as well as food for animals – so GHG are only one of many negative consequences. Additionally, the once-eccentric prospect of lab-grown meat as an appropriate intervention is exciting to hear about, especially as it gains momentum. My final point is that caring for the environment and eating meat do not have to be mutually exclusive.

THE RATIONAL SOUL

Hierocles was a Stoic who was described as a "holy man". Scholars know little about Hierocles except for his influential book *Elements of Ethics*, in which he discusses self-perception. He talks about animals from the moment of their birth having a constant self-perception; this perception being the most basic faculty of animals. This is based on *oikeiôsis*, a Greek term to do with belonging to the self, roughly translating to "affinity", or "appropriation". *Oikeiôsis* includes the concept that good is exclusive to rational beings – the relevant point being that animals are not considered rational.

This concept of the Stoics was similar to the position Aristotle (384 BC – 322 BC) held. In his book *Metaphysics* he defined "human" as the rational animal and therefore rejects the idea that another species could be rational. Donald Robertson, who made his way through various excerpts of the Stoics (specifically Epictetus, Marcus and Seneca), came to the conclusion that living creatures could be divided into three categories: "wild", "domestic" and "rational" animals. Rational animals, as Aristotle believed, are explicitly adult humans who are capable of wisdom and virtue. "Wild" animals, such as wolves, tigers and hyenas are savage and passionate – these are beasts which wish to do nothing but bite and act violent through their untamed nature. Finally we have the "domestic" animals, such as cattle, sheep or horses, which are irrational, and as Mr Robertson says, "are concerned mainly with their fodder".

Aristotle and Plato both reject that the non-rational soul of a child is transformed and then replaced by the rational soul as they grow older. But it appears that the standard Stoic view was that children, as well as animals, are irrational. But of course there's a difference between them, as Diogenes Laërtius says: "Reason intervenes as the craftsman of impulse." The crucial point here is that children have the potential – fate permitting – to become a craftsman.

To counter this you may propose the argument that if the value of the life of a being is determined by its capability of a rational thought, would that reasoning extend to people with mental illness and intellectual disabilities? Or to any people who cannot sustain themselves or express any kind of rational thought? Or does that only apply to animals? This point is a strong argument.

Some may side with the idea that this special status of the human is all that needs to be argued for. Others may side with the idea that pain defines rationality and so eating fish is perfectly acceptable, or that animals were put on this earth for us to consume as seen in Cicero's account of Chrysippus' view in *On the Nature of the Gods*. But many of these ideas are false. For example, fish very evidently do have nociceptors (responsible for signalling pain). Evolutionary biologist and author Richard Dawkins has argued that less intelligent animals feel more pain. They would need more pain to signal to their brains that they are in trouble; whereas a human only needs slight pain to contemplate what could happen with more exposure to this pain.

TEMPERATE EATING

Rejecting pleasures such as eating a tasty food is an acknowledgement of its power over you. This can create a situation where we treat these foods as tempting desires. This temptation creates tension, and this tension has to be released at some point. We can compare this to Cynic philosophy where restriction from pleasure becomes the pathway to happiness or the "shortcut to virtue", an attitude which I believe is aligned towards the very strict and extreme dietary plans that are known to be ineffective long term. There's a subtle but important difference between self-control and self-deprivation. Stoicism allows for some leeway, as long as the agenda remains congruent and your mind unattached to the occasional sweet. I believe it is worth having planned and controlled "refeed" or "cheat" days, for the psychological release of tension to allow more flexibility in your nutrition.

According to the journal *Metabolism*, an all-out binge will only increases one's metabolic rate by 3–10 per cent for approximately one day. This is the equivalent to 200–500 calories, so think about how much food you'd need to eat to achieve that effect. Let's say you'd need 600 calories; then on a typical refeed day, you will be at maintenance calories or in a surplus. Of course, if we are counting calories on a weekly basis this doesn't make that much of a difference to long-term practice. The point is that refeed days aren't effective enough metabolically to pursue out of direct physiological effects. Increasing your calories may flush water from under the skin, perhaps then giving the illusion of being leaner. Similarly to a low-carbohydrate diet, certain effects of increasing your calories periodically give immediate visible change.

A healthy man can help others better and for longer. Antonius the Pious (AD 86–161), one of the truly great Roman Emperors, kept a simple diet so he could work from dawn to dusk with as few bathroom interruptions as possible. He did this in order to be at the service of the people for longer. The less time you put into your workouts, but the more effort, the greater the reward. The less time we are focused on exercise and correcting our nutrition, the more time we can spend on our philosophy. Our "keen edge", Seneca said, is too often dulled by heavy eating and then wasted further as we drain our life force in exercise trying to work it off. Simply put, your diet is more important than the exercises you do and must be your first priority.

To quote Musonius Rufus: "And indeed at each meal, there is not one hazard for going wrong, but many. First of all, the man who eats more than he ought does wrong, and also the man who wallows in the pickles and sauces, and the man who prefers the sweeter foods to the more healthful ones, and the man who does not serve food of the same kind or amount to his guests as to himself."

There are certain factors which are mostly out of our control, such as the pollution we breathe in walking to work or the chemicals in our water system. So it's important to recognise where our food comes from. As researcher Catherine Shanahan puts it: "Food is less like a fuel and more like a language conveying information." Her point is that if you eat a steak from a grass-fed cow, you shouldn't only be concerned with how the food is cooked, what it looks like, etc. You should also consider where the cow was from, what the cow ate (which grasses), even as far as knowing the quality of the soil which the grass grew in. Shanahan says food is like a language, and this language of the food source is spoken and communicated to the body as we consume it. Perhaps the comprehension rate could be analogous to health. The way I see this analogy being understood is to see the best decision (perhaps choosing grass-fed meat) as correct spelling and grammar of the language.

Tasting something is studying it. Through your taste buds you direct the information of the food and then you come to a conclusion. You recognise certain flavours that appeal to you, others that don't; you feel the texture of the food and experience its fragrance and aroma. Similar to a scientific study, there's an aim, hypothesis, results, discussion and finally a conclusion.

If you are educating yourself to more expensive palates you may mourn the loss of ability to enjoy simple pleasures such as an apple or potato with no added sauces. Why would anyone wish to regularly enjoy expensive food in the first place? Is there some sort of elation felt as a consequence of spending more money on sophisticated food? Musonius speaks of people's appetites needing to be "sharpened" through wine, vinegar and tart sauces. When I speak of appetite in this context it isn't only feeling hungry but also the willingness of an individual to eat when full. Musonius believes those who have picky tendencies use sauces to spice up their food in order to make it more appealing and be able to eat and increase their desire for the food. The more expensive your palate becomes the more this depends on what is out of your control. You may find yourself questioning why you should attempt to eat food which is cheap, simple, and healthy when an expensive palate is within one's resources. Once you adjust yourself to an expensive taste it can become difficult to take pride in your enjoyment of simple food.

Seneca tells us that although "water, barley meal, and crusts of barley bread, are not a cheerful diet, yet it is the highest kind of pleasure to be able to derive pleasure from this sort of food". As previously mentioned, it would appear that Musonius was correct in advocating for plain food. Plain food, with fewer spices and less sauce would naturally have a less potent fragrance. Nature itself provided a palate which calibrates the response of smell. The best foods aren't the most expensive; they are the fundamental foods found in nature. Use simple, basic and easy recipes, not only to appreciate the taste of simplicity but also to exercise frugality.

Musonius, like Socrates, advises that we must *eat to live, while a foolish man lives to eat.* In the past the rich were fat and the poor were thin; today it is quite the opposite. The rich are now thin and the poor are fat! Perhaps the frugal mindset is now obsolete. Wide empirical evidence shows us that children and adults from low socio-economic groups are more likely to be obese in the Western world. This doesn't mean that cheap and healthy food doesn't exist, though. It does mean that more care is needed in order to spend money wisely. An example of this in my own life is going to the farmers' market early Sunday morning instead of the supermarket later in the day. Seneca further advises what a noble soul must do, saying that: "To descend of one's own free will to a diet which even those who have been sentenced to death have not to fear! This is indeed forestalling the spear thrusts of Fortune."

Archaeologist Eugenia Salza Prina Ricotti wrote the fascinating book *Meals and Recipes from Ancient Greece*. Most of the recipes in the book are derived from a single text written by

Athenaeus, who was a Greek rhetorician and grammarian. His book *Deipnosophists* (which means "dinner-table philosophers"), gave Ms Ricotti the idea for her book. This is somewhat unrelated to the ideas we are covering but I had to find some way to include this as it is a book I urge you keep in your kitchen.

In the book Ms Ricotti presents a recipe called Zeno's lentil soup. Apparently Zeno was fond of a soup made from leeks, carrots, vinegar, honey and coriander. It's ironic that Zeno was fed lentil soup by his teachers in order to cure him of his modesty. Lentil soup for the Cynics was a common symbol and expression of their values, which Zeno was largely influenced by. Start here in the book and try the soup out, it's a simple recipe and I actually made it recently in celebration of finishing this book – although the recipe was disappointing as there was no sage.

The Mediterranean diet has long been symbolic of good health. For example, the Sardinian people (who live on an island in Italy) live to very old ages. Sardinia is located in one of a few "blue zones" of the world. (A "blue zone" is an area where it is common for people to live healthy lives into their 90s or beyond.) The Sardinians eat lava beans, barley, goats' milk, tomatoes and Cannonau wine, as well as olive oil and mostly plant-based foods. They are extremely active and have some of the highest numbers of people living over 100 years old. The ancients ate similar foods to this modern diet.

Within the city of Athens vegetables were actually quite expensive and the poorer class ate dried vegetables. Lentil soup was a very typical dish for the workman. Legumes and cereals were common too, as well as grains such as wheat, oat and barley. Olive oil and red wine were common in both Greece and Rome. Goats' and sheep's milk were also seen as superior compared to cow's milk – which is actually what the science supports today. Meat was not a common food for the majority and was eaten during festivals (usually religious), and as a luxury for the upper class.

MOTIVES IN COGNITIVE MODELLING

"Your attempt was always subject to reservations, remember; you were not aiming at the impossible. At what, then? Simply at making the attempt itself. In this you succeeded; and with that the object of your existence is attained."

– Marcus Aurelius

The neurotransmitter dopamine is the dominant chemical in the inner workings of the brain's reward system. Dopamine plays a critical role in cognition, motivation and emotions, and is known mostly for its contribution to our feelings of reward and pleasure, although one misconception is that it is responsible for pleasure itself. Rather it is the driver of the reward cycle which involves pleasurable stimuli. Having sex, eating and other instruments of stimuli all play on the release of dopamine. Pleasure that comes from these natural stimuli reinforces our inclination to go back to these stimuli, as they are central to our survival through our biologically driven purpose to procreate ("calories into babies" was the term I once heard). It's noteworthy that despite differences in how certain stimuli affect us, all pleasurable dependencies work on a very similar mechanism of triggering the dopaminergic activity in the brain. You may notice that when somebody quits one destructive habit, multiple other successes follow.

Food is a reinforcer of dopamine and essentially out-competes other behaviours. Perhaps this explains why obesity remains such a prominent problem, yet is more socially accepted than other dependencies (drugs, cigarettes, etc.). If someone consumed sugar in excess, this would result in the recurrent release of abnormal levels of dopamine. Prolonged exposure of the synaptic cleft (the gap where neurons meet and neurotransmitters diffuse) results in a down regulation of a specific neural pathway. When down regulation of mesolimbic dopamine receptors occurs there is an evident decrease in the naturally occurring sensitivity to the exposure of the specific stimuli.

The average human has thousands of words stored in their vocabulary available for speech. With that many words there are so many thoughts which can be conjured at one single moment. Yet we think about such specific thoughts and desires and focus immensely on the details surrounding them. You stretch, you yawn, you peek through the window to see whether it's a sunny day. Thirty minutes later, something starts to signal hunger in your brain, and you start to crave the taste of salty and the texture of crunchy. This salty-crunchy food is rationalised through imagination and your previous memory – towards French fries. When this motive comes into your brain, leptin, known as the satiety hormone (produced by adipose, or fat, tissue), binds to the receptors of the hypothalamus region in the brain. The hypothalamus is also associated with certain dependencies of certain drugs.

Let's say this hunger signal comes when you are preparing documents for today's work. Your hypothalamus will keep firing this signal over and over until this notifier becomes the identity you crave to embody. You remember what it's like to desire this food. The more you remember, the more you become infatuated with your future self being fulfilled by the satisfaction associated with eating French fries. At this moment, the thought will become so distracting that you will stand up and begin a nondeterministic behavioural momentum towards the objective, therefore submitting to the motive French fries. Professor Jordan Peterson describes this idea like an animal chasing its prey. The chase is nondeterministic in the sense that you may choose to buy fast food instead of cooking your own.

You may presume that satiation (when the motive is fulfilled) is the pleasure, but it is not. This is a common misconception of our society. The understanding of *when* pleasure is felt is what distinguishes the temperate and the moderate from those individuals with a disposition to dependency and attachment. The chase, the voyage, the search – this is what arouses excitement. It is in this search that we live; it is this chase which arouses the desire for French fries in the first place. If it was not the search itself which subconsciously gave rise to the motive then we would all surely die, as satiation would never occur. If the search wasn't the pleasure then in Palaeolithic times humans would have had a disinterest in actually hunting.

This behavioural phenomenon is commonly found in those working on a project, such as writing a book, but never actually finishing it. It's not that these individuals lack the cognitive capability; it's quite the opposite. The truth lies in their deep arousal of the journey itself. Once the book, health goal, weight, whatever is achieved, true pleasure is missing. It is replaced by satisfaction. This satisfaction, although enjoyable in its own right, reveals the depth of the void carved out by the search. Now, this principle is to your advantage if you acknowledge its existence. On the other hand, if ignorant, it is a societal narrative which deludes the layman into embracing satiation as the pleasure. Going back to a more micro scale (food), after satiation your hypothalamus must create a new persona.

Seneca says, "Show me a man who isn't a slave…one is a slave to sex, another to money, another to ambition; all are slaves to hope or fear." We are all slaves to this search as it is what maintains life itself. I think this desire for satiation resurfaces more quickly after a food like French fries, especially if purchased as fast food. Simply swiping your credit card exacerbates the emptiness post-satiation. The chase becomes very short, and this is the only true pleasurable component. This is the reason behind binge eating. Even after a person is full and the food doesn't taste good any more, the person continues to eat. The length of the chase shortens more and more. Years ago, the lengthy search (hunting and gathering) lasted for hours or even days at a time, and it is in this search where we lived.

This is simply another affirmation for the food culture we find in Italy and France.

To summarise:

- As an individual is introduced to natural food they experience reasonable "pleasure".

- As they are introduced to processed food, this "pleasure" increases dramatically.

- As they become used to this unnaturally high "pleasure", the body rejects natural food.

- As unnatural food is repeatedly reintroduced again, the "pleasure" no longer satisfies the anticipated high.

- More is eaten to fill in the void of lost satiation, and true pleasure decreases.

The moral of the story here is that we must try to extend the period of true pleasure, rather than focus on the chase, and solidify this period as habit and a priority. As Epictetus said: "Whatever you would make habitual, practise it; and if you would not make it habitual, do not practise it, but habituate yourself to something else."

"But if thought corrupts language, language can also corrupt thought"

– George Orwell.

REFRAMING YOUR IDENTITY

In life we all have certain identities or personas we attach ourselves to. For example, a heavy smoker has identified smoking as a part of his character. We often define ourselves by what we experience through our senses – our pleasures, our routines. They come together to form a contemporary persona. You can't deny that habits have at least *some* influence on your character. To shift out of the identity of being a smoker or a food connoisseur requires permanent change. Changing your identity may be seen as your ability to restrict yourself, hold off from temptation and restrain the urge to submit to pleasure – but this is wrong. It may seem that restraint is the only means to change a habit, but remember the habit is based on your identity, not the thing itself.

There's a major flaw in this idea of restriction and restraint; it is a short-term pursuit and will again build tension which will be released at some point. When this release occurs, it can become more difficult to bounce back and try again. As Epictetus tells us: "Men are disturbed, not by things, but by the principles and notions which they form concerning things." Bad habits weigh us down on our journey to moral excellence; like an anchor they can pull us back. It's our job to untie each anchor one at a time in order to quicken our ascent.

This verbal-behavioural idea is expressed well through the results of a 2012 study published in the *Journal of Consumer Research*. Researchers offered participants a chocolate bar (unhealthy option) or a granola bar (perceived healthier option) to thank them for their time. One group was asked to use the phrase "I don't" before instigating their refusal to the temptation and the other group was asked to use the phrase "I can't". Thirty-nine per cent of people who used "I can't" picked the healthier option, while 64 per cent who said "I don't" picked the healthy option.

Writer Oliver Burkeman tells us, "The 'can't' framing implies an external restraint, which feels disempowering (even if you imposed the restraint on yourself)...To say that you 'don't' do something, by contrast, suggests autonomy, as well as long-term commitment." It's very clear that to resist a temptation and eliminate the chance of it happening you must say "no". What the *Journal of Consumer Research* study shows is that the manner in which you say "no" has crucial implications. Using "I can't" is the same as saying "I quit smoking". When offered a cigarette and you say "I can't" you are affirming the fact that this is a struggle for you and in due course every time you say these words you are reaffirming that it takes *effort* for you to resist the urge. This implies that you will inevitably fail. However, when you say "I don't" you are actively shifting the paradigm of how you define yourself. Every single time you say "I don't" it's empowering in the sense that it's cumulative. The more you say "I don't" the more you embody this.

When I was in France I saw so many young people smoking. What surprised me was the number of young women who smoked. To a few, I posed the question: "Why do you smoke?" They replied in a joking manner, "Well, you know, I'm French." Although it may sound like a joke, people underestimate the power of social narratives in dictating the direction of their life. When I briefly lived in Canada I experienced the narrative construct of smoking being extremely "uncool". This specific narrative says you should/shouldn't smoke and so a majority follows it. The extent of a narrative holding power of people's objectivity is frightening and likewise empowering. The philosopher Martin Heidegger framed this as denying death, telling us that: "Every man is born as many men and dies as a single one".

Marcus Aurelius said: "You have power over your own mind – not outside events. Realise this, and you will find strength." The happiness of your life is simply a representation of the quality of your thoughts; nothing more, nothing less. This implies that it is possible to reframe any situation we are experiencing into a good one, even if it appears to be bad. When you are stuck in the paradigm of "I'm a smoker" or "I eat junk food and that's what I do", you are reinforcing the normalcy of it "just being who you are".

These thoughts are the problem; they exacerbate the anguish within you, despite objective awareness of self-degeneration. You may find yourself accepting and embracing normalcy as a way to comfort the ego and your natural inclination to seek some sort of comfortable regime. Discomfort provokes uncertainty, and discomfort is all you have when you are reduced to shifting a characteristic that has solidified within you. The notion of changing and experiencing discomfort becomes everything your ego wishes to resist and everything your truest self wishes to become, and this creates conflict. This antagonism manifests as the carefree nihilistic slant many have towards their addictions. The classic example is a smoker who is shown factual proof that smoking will kill him, or sees the horrifying images on the packet of cigarettes of the diseases he is bringing upon himself – and yet still he opens the box and proceeds to light ten cigarettes that day.

> "It is not because things are difficult that we do not dare, it is because we do not dare that they are difficult."
>
> – Seneca

There is considerable evidence suggesting that mesolimbic dopamine pathway is the cause for the craving that people experience towards these objective negative behaviours. The final conscious decision to make a wrong decision comes from emotional processing through the inner workings of dopamine, but prior to this decision being made there are environmental factors which can provoke the given emotive responses. Creating an environment around you that supports the changes you wish you to make is vital for your success. This can come through a change in language as previously mentioned, but also in the way you prioritise the social and logistical aspects of your life.

What we eat every single day is largely attributed to what we're presented with. Now, don't get me wrong – the individual who chooses to eat the food is at fault and anybody who has gotten out of shape did that to themselves. But we should still respect the power of external forces, such as environment, in governing the likelihood of an emotional decision being acted upon. This is closely related to the psychological phenomenon of acting and behaving in a similar manner to those around you, as the saying goes: "You are the average of the five people you spend the most time with." This idea is not exclusive to your success financially and socially; the people around you have direct influence on your health and well-being, which is why it's not uncommon to see entire families obese.

You must surround yourself with people who mirror the direction you want to head in, or at the very least, with a wider variety of people so that it is less likely you become influenced by those with bad habits. This doesn't mean you need to isolate yourself from people in your life; just make sure you spend the appropriate amount of time with the people who are and aren't emulating your highest character. As Epictetus tells us: "Every creature is naturally formed to flee and abhor things that appear hurtful and that which causes them; and to pursue and admire those which appear beneficial and that which causes them." But remember that just because you're not particularly fond of someone, this doesn't mean that their critiques, albeit potentially harsh are necessarily wrong. Don't let your ego ignore what may be true in spite of your opinion of the individual.

Remind yourself of the virtue and moral goodness of others. Think about the modesty of one friend, the honesty of another, another's commitment to their well-being and any other good quality of another man, and you will find your own good. Marcus Aurelius reminds us that "nothing delights so much as the examples of virtues", and we must keep them surrounding us at all times. Furthermore, understand that habits are triggered by normalcy. For instance, if you have the habit of smoking after eating a large meal, or eat sugar when you are stressed, you must become very aware of the relationship between these habits. The more you're aware the more you'll simply understand what you do, when you do it and what provoked you to do it. Objectively we know what's good for us; therefore it can be extremely frustrating to understand the harm you are inflicting upon yourself and likewise know what the pragmatic solutions are. To the spectator the solution is practical and self-explanatory, nonsensical, possibly even absurd. "Stop smoking!" others will tell you. "Stop eating so much, exercise more." This is like telling somebody who has no job to take paid leave.

Temptation will arise when we are trying to shift into a more favourable lifestyle. It is how we deal with these temptations that determines whether the act is accomplished successfully. The longer we remain indifferent to these temptations over time the easier it becomes to do so, and the more we can desensitise ourselves to their appearance. They may never disappear but we can train ourselves to keep walking through them as they come. Understand *why* you want to stop in the first place, always remembering that *eudaimonia* (peace of mind) is true human joy. Focus on the fact that if you do overcome a dependency you will likely become a better person and experience more *eudaimonia*. *Eudaimonia* is without a doubt worth the temporary struggle you may need to endure.

Finally, remember that all dependencies are related in some way or the other, just as language is. So start small, or start big – just remember to start. French is related to English, and although Mandarin and German may be further apart, they are all still languages. So learn one language and others become easier to pick up.

Redesigning the Brain

I know what it's like to be helpless at the mercy of an external force in your life so conflicting from your deepest self, but yet so familiar and comforting to you. Many of our most difficult pursuits in life aren't necessarily our careers and successes – they are the personal battles against addictions, depression and other internal antagonists (which most human beings experience to some extent).

Although there are various means which provide us with short-term relief, which can be therapeutic and useful, permanent change should always be the objective. It is unwise to place long-term *eudaimonia* on a variable which is replaceable, fragile, external and thus temporary. You as an individual have the capacity to change the direction you head in. Our brain is extremely malleable and adaptive and has the potential for mass change. This change is difficult; but it is also very possible to do with the right programming.

Depression is a state of feeling sad and in despair (not be confused with a typical change in moods). In ancient times the word *melancholy* was used, which is a more holistic description of ailments which also included obsession, fear and anger. Anger is something the Stoics wrote a lot about. It was described as a temporary madness. Depression is more long term and can affect your concentration, hinder your ability to rationalise and disturb your sleeping patterns, in a manner which genuinely feels endless and inescapable. I think very depressed people love the depressed state; it's realistic, it's comfortable, it's a foundation they can always rely on and this love grows with time.

A friend once asked me, "Do you think one can be content in misery?" My reply was yes and I think one *should* be. Suffering is nature's framework, so "content" could mean either you embrace moral badness in response to this framework of misery, or you are content with the reality of it and strive for moral excellence. There is no escaping being content with misery; the significance is in the response.

To most, happiness is sought after in order to compensate for the dissonance one experiences, instead of simply being accepted for what it is and welcomed through its natural abundance. Just as marketing is based on what people *want* to hear as opposed to true objective reality, so is our own personal basis for virtue. Contemporary self-help literature is reflective of this idea, accomplishing little more than providing persuasive yet redundant rhetoric on the importance of "positive thinking". Don't mistake my critique of this literature as a testimony to my distaste with positive thinking, as this is far from the case. The positivity movement is flawed because much of its advice seeks to escape the reality that most of our lives *are* full of suffering. I urge you to entertain the idea that your misery is *not the point*. We must embrace a measure of suffering to live *correctly* rather than deluding ourselves into the comfort of cyclical and useless tracking of the momentary judgements of how happy we feel.

An animal's primary instinctual behaviour is to live, to self-preserve. This is an impulse given by nature from the very beginning of life. In the book *On Ends*, Chrysippus explains to us that the most treasured objective of every animal is simply the existence it knows, more specifically its awareness of this existence. Do you ever see an animal disassociate from itself, or distance from itself its own conscious preservation? Because of this natural autonomy of self-preservation, we must then assert that nature gives an attraction to what is good for the animal, and opposition to what holds potential injury and harm. The universal governing force must be harmonious. When virtue is upheld then a man is happy.

Cleanthes asserts to us that happiness is essentially a disposition of the mind, meaning that the mind is consistently in harmony. What we may frequently come to see as inconsistency is the external; the external is deceitful, the external does nothing but influence our associations. We are indoctrinated our whole lives with the false belief that we can achieve happiness through acquisition – but the reality of consistent harmony being abundant as an available source seems impossible.

Many see depression as an entity of its own. The truth of the matter is that yes, it can be genetic for many; but people tend to underestimate the influence of *choices* on the presence of this lingering sadness. In certain cases, there are people who have chemical deficiencies in their brain, but much of a depressed state can be re-regulated through changes in habits. For some, perhaps this won't work, but this doesn't exclude the merit of trying everything possible before an antidepressant is used. A depressive state may lessen your ability to focus on the health and strength of your body, but the chemical response of the brain can somewhat be seen as an external force and one that we cannot necessarily control right now. Out diet is also important for this. The idea of fish consumption relative to rates of depression has been known for a while. Countries such as New Zealand, Australia and the United States have low consumption of fish and high depression, while Japan has the highest amount and the least depression according to a 2015 meta-analysis by the *Journal of Epidemiology & Community Health*. However, there are two problems with this. Firstly, it's population based, meaning it's not causative, and secondly, there's a chance that societal norms about the expression of depression are different in Japan compared to New Zealand. Regardless, we know very evidently that the fatty acids in fish as well as other foods alleviate cognitive disorders.

What we can control is our reaction to these ailments. Living in accordance to nature isn't going to be defined by how healthy you are despite your depression, it's going to be defined by your effort to control your reaction to it and do the best that you can. Being healthy is not virtue; virtue is the attempt to live in accordance to the actions which often precede these results. Marcus Aurelius explains it this way: "Our inward power, when it obeys nature, reacts to events by accommodating itself to what it faces – to what is possible. It needs no specific material. It pursues its own aims as circumstances allow; it turns obstacles into fuel, as a fire overwhelms what would have quenched a lamp. What's thrown on top of the conflagration is absorbed, consumed by it – and makes it burn still higher."

We can plan a diet in order to lose weight, and maybe you will be fortunate enough to pursue your goals uninterrupted. Perhaps you will be lucky enough to never meet obstacles. If you haven't realised yet, I'm not here to sell you the best cure or market the "ultimate secret". I'm being the unpopular realist here and revealing to you the long-awaited secret: your circumstances and your willingness to pursue the discomforts that come your way are what will bring you success.

If I were to ask you whether the very best businesses are those which are most popular, you may answer along the lines of, "Well, of course they are. Clearly they are offering a high value point and based on the product or service they provide, a larger proportion of people are inclined to support this business due to its respective quality." You could also apply the same question and argument to political campaigns and the relationship of the quality of results to the number of voters these campaigns pull in. Now the latter example isn't necessarily *wrong*, but the truth is that in more cases than you would expect these campaigns or popularised businesses may be leaning towards the more irrational.

FREEDOM IN THE MARKETPLACE

Business people and politicians sit around all day long coming up with methods to market and feed you the information you *want* to hear. In fact, if a politician or a business person came to you in order to solve an issue and logically gave you the complex reality behind a problem, then undoubtedly you would be less inclined to support them, as there is far more opportunity for you to find fault in their message. I may veer slightly off topic here, but stay with me…

People say that *The Simpsons* predicted the election of Donald Trump. I say it was Socrates. Democracy has long been seen as a good thing. A democratic country is symbolic of fairness, honesty and honour. However, we must think about whether it is fair that any ordinary person is free to make an influential judgement on who should be the ruler of a country. Socrates told us that voting should be seen as more of a skill, rather than a right given to any breathing citizen. This may sound like an argument for elitism, but it's not. Socrates held the belief that only those who think deeply and rationally about the relevant issue should be given the right to cast a vote. His fear was that a completely free democracy would lead to demagoguery – that is, appealing to emotion rather than to reasoned thought.

Trump's iconic "make America great again" slogan was an example of demagoguery, because it appealed to voters' emotions. He could have said: "America will be a greater nation if we do X and Y, because of Z consequence." Don't take this as disdain of Donald Trump himself. Instead, take this as questioning the system which allowed a reality TV star to rise to power; and likewise the power of the layman to sell programmes and products that are clearly ineffective. I understand the latter example seems slightly off topic, but take into consideration the following examples. You've probably come across these, or something like them, before.

"The four-minute abs programme!"

"The one-week water-fasting cleanse!"

"Buy this program and you will lose thirty pounds in ten days or your money back – with a sixty-day guarantee!"

And you think to yourself: "What a bargain; what's the harm in trying? I mean, everyone else is talking about it."

Then the rational side of your brain starts questioning: "Hey, are you sure about this?"

But that's drowned out by the non-rational side of your brain: "They are on television and have the financial capacity to advertise themselves over and over, so how on earth could this be false? I mean, sure, perhaps they are somewhat exaggerating – so I'll lose twenty-eight pounds in ten days, not thirty. But I'm happy with that."

Think about a course, a product, a book, a diet or nutritional plan that promises big results. If any one of these was actually exceptional, it would require people to actually *think* in order utilise and make use of it. This reason is exactly why the diets and fat-loss pills that don't work rise to the top even though objectively they are *not* the best option. The market is a free-for-all, with people's insecurities giving greedy companies the ability to take advantage of people's emotional compulsions. Worst of all, we shrug our shoulders and accept it.

Now, in no way am I attempting to boast about my writing; neither am I trying to say that this is an exceptional piece of work. However, I give no simple step-by-step guide or short-term and short-cut system which is guaranteed to work no matter what, and this is the reason why I am adamant *The Stoic Body* will never be a mainstream book. But I am content, so long as the few reading these words understand reality and begin to rejoice in thinking on a deeper level, on a higher plain of consciousness. Forget short cuts; strive to emulate processes which are more difficult and take longer, but are clearly the most fruitful and rewarding options.

You should *consider* (but only consider and not blindly follow) eating vegetables and natural foods and following a certain method of exercise. The key is to not compare yourself to others to the point where you discourage yourself from pursuing an alternative (which may possibly be more optimal for your individual circumstances). To give an example, the use of psilocybin mushrooms is a means to quit an addiction, with a remarkable 80 per cent or more success rate in the long-term. This is not a Stoic practice per se, as Stoicism generally advocates for sobriety. This is an unorthodox example which evidence is surprisingly supporting more and more in recent years, and I thought it would be interesting to mention, because, well...why not.

Naturally, the next question is: "Who should I trust with advice, when there are so many resources out there, many of which are conflicting and confusing?" Should you trust the most qualified, the most gifted, the most competent in the act itself? These attributes all have merit and of course they should be taken into consideration for very specific questions regarding injury and disease but there is a greater judgement you can use to make your decisions. Ask yourself these questions:

Would you take the advice of somebody naturally gifted

at painting, or somebody who was average, but with years of effort, failure and even harsh criticism became as good as the person naturally gifted?

What can I change? If I can change this, will the act submit me to obsessional passion or will these acts be virtuous, exclusive of the goal? (Through answering this question you will find what you *can* change and whether you *should* change it.)

Is the man offering the programme, book, whatever it is that you're interested in, living a life which is of just or unjust nature? If just, consider the advice; if unjust, use it as an example of what *not* to do.

Writer and politician Niccolò Machiavelli says: "The armour of others is too wide, or too straight for us; it falls off us; or it weighs us down." What Machiavelli means is that what works for some doesn't for others. Your decision should be based on exposing yourself to as many different sources as. Only take advice from yourself – but only if you have entered into an "abundance framed mentality". An abundance framed mentality means that you have exposed yourself to multiple options and sources and so you're pulling your guidance from abundance rather than scarcity, often referred to as a scarcity mindset.

Even if your efforts suffice and you are able to cut out a bad habit for the short term, this doesn't mean you have finished. You're never finished; your peace of mind comes from your constant and determined attempts to be free of dependence, which is never achieved. The multi-billion dollar health and self-help industry thrives off the misfortune of human insecurity and vulnerability. I don't mean to be pessimistic and blame the industry for the troubles people face. I just want you to understand without any doubt that all the empowerment you require is within *you* and your mindset, *not* a supplement which most likely is a placebo and wastes your money.

What I've learned through my life is that often confronting

temptation and understanding how to work pleasure is much like a conversation.

First, ask yourself the question: "What is the nature of this pleasure?" You must guard against being carried away by the power pleasure can have over you. There is a very subtle pause that must be recognised in the brief seconds prior to an emotion-based act taking place. Think about those who intentionally pause in a spoken sentence; this is done in order to add power and substance to their verbal acuity. Similarly, you must delay your acts from your thoughts in order to give your "little spark of rationality" the chance to enforce itself. You must think of both times: the time where you are going to enjoy the pleasure for what it is, and the other time, after the satiation, where, as Seneca says: "You will repent and will reproach yourself." If you are to undertake the thing, you have to be aware of the charm and also be aware that it shall not conquer you. Always keep in mind how much better it is that you have gained the victory of pausing and therefore avoiding the experience of repent and reproach.

You can pause in the emotional moment between a decision, and create tension and power in your interaction, just as you can in conversation. You're less likely to dismiss similar moments in the future as being insignificant when you extend the seconds in this pause. First impressions count and it can be difficult to revoke first impressions, whether you come to like a person or not. You've most likely experienced this yourself. If someone lies when you first meet them you'll always see them as a liar; if someone makes you laugh on first impression you will likely see this person as the humorous type.

Imagine your future encounters with a food or any substance (which you know you would enjoy) and imagine it as meeting a new person – you want to give off the best first impression to essentially set the stage for the rest of the relationship.

PART THREE:
REHEARSING POVERTY

"My dear Lucilius, you will leap for joy when filled with a pennyworth of food, and you will understand that a man's peace of mind does not depend upon Fortune; for, even when angry she grants enough for our needs."

– Seneca

THE HOMEOSTATIC IDEAL

You've probably heard of "calories in and calories out" as a response to "I can't lose weight". The solution advocated is usually to eat less and exercise more. This is true – but only to a point.

Many people (even trainers) treat calories in/calories out as the solution to people's fat loss, but in that case, anyone with the ability to do basic arithmetic would be a top-class fat-loss coach – right? You're always losing fat and gaining fat at the same time, but what's important is which beats the other over time.

Firstly, there's a difference between weight loss and fat loss

– a big difference. To lose weight (which could mean muscle or fat) you need to have burned more calories than you have expended. The same applies to fat loss, sure, but there's a much greater emphasis on the macronutrients which you are taking in as a means to determine how much or how little muscle you retain. For example, you need slightly more protein when in a caloric deficit to preserve your muscle mass.

We know that some foods don't digest as well as others, and some people's digestive systems are not good at absorbing fat, therefore leaving them in danger of not having enough fat available for basic metabolic functions. We also have to consider an individual's genes and how their hormones (cortisol, DHEA, growth hormone, insulin), and other critical factors such as sleep and exercise, work for their body. Calories in versus calories *metabolised* is a better way to express it, in my opinion. However, despite what you hear about various theories on calories "not counting", understand that regardless, wide empirical evidence makes it very clear consistent energy balance determines body weight. Macronutrients as well as other variables such as sleep and exercises complicate exactly what is being lost or gained.

TRACKING CALORIES

The most reliable source is to just track the intake of food. Measure changes in your body weight (same circumstances) over, let's say three weeks. From here, calculate the change in body weight. If it's 2 kg in a week or 0 kg, this will tell you whether you're on the right track. This self-referencing and tracking of weight and food intake isn't the best way to secure sustainability and longevity, but it is a great start.

Progression in fat loss is never going to be linear, even though we wish it to be. For instance, an individual who weighs 100 kg will lose weight at a different rate to an individual who weighs 65 kg, as they are losing a different proportion of their weight (analogous to how we experience time more rapidly as we age). An interesting study in 2010 by the *International Journal of Behavioral Medicine* shows that in obese populations more aggressive caloric restriction is positively associated with long-term success. I would suspect that this has a large psychological basis – a change in mindset, for instance.

What often happens is stagnation and a break of linear progress, more commonly referred to as a plateau. Plateaus can be divided into two categories. The first is a plateau where your body has actually stopped progressing; the second is where you perceive the body to have stopped progressing. Despite the negative connotation you may attach to a plateau, I encourage you, as I do my clients, to simply see this as a natural part of your progression, rather than a hindrance. A plateau is simply showing you that you are taking action.

The *set point theory* was originally coined by researchers William Bennett and Joel Gurin as a means to explain why dieting is so ineffective in giving people long-lasting changes in their physical composition. The idea is that the body defends a certain range of body weight (and body fat in particular). Think of set point theory as a constant feedback loop in your body, revolving around a homeostatic ideal. It is a fact that our bodies maintain an optimal weight very closely, according to a study in 2000 from *Nature* and another in 2004 from the *Diabetes & Metabolism* journal – both of which concluded the significance of genetic and heritable variables on body weight regulation.

Environmental factors such as nutrition, hormones (stress and appetite), exercise (frequency and intensity) are also important. Studies show us that there's a significant relationship between appetite and levels of energy conservation. The body is regulated asymmetrically, meaning that we are more effective when active in response to weight loss, rather than weight gain. When the metabolism is slowed down, the level of hunger rises as movement lessens. When rats are given an abundance of food they very rapidly get pulled back to their previously defended homeostatic set point. Many people fall back to their old weight. Evidence for the set point theory has shown us that this isn't necessarily just because of habits; rather this homeostatic comfort zone and asymmetric physiology makes a set point to settle on very appealing for the body. This can be a frustrating and grim concept to wrap your head around.

A meta-analysis exploring successful weight-loss maintenance from the *Annual Review of Nutrition* in 2001 showed us that the best outcome for any weight-loss programme is regaining 77 per cent of the initial weight lost by the fourth or fifth years. In the meta-analysis, less than 50 per cent of those enrolled were actually able to achieve this result (which really isn't much) while the remaining subjects gained over 77 per cent of the initial weight lost.

What is even more convincing is that most who try to adjust their set point and lose weight fail within two years. It's difficult to change your set point; but you can change your weight within the parameters of your natural set point, especially by building muscle.

Certain weights and appearances become correlated to ideal health, which unfortunately form a standard that doesn't reflect true health, as this is subjective to the set point of many. Natural variations of set points are often argued to be excluded from the socially constructed range, and this poses issues and conflict. Perhaps this is why we find it so difficult to permanently shift out of a certain weight category, not only physiologically but also psychologically. When we have an issue which is evident in both these spheres of the human condition then it's difficult to combat. Please keep in mind this isn't to argue in favour of the very delusional belief that you can be healthy at any weight (I'd be the last to ever support such a form of activism).

The point here is that this should all come back to focusing on virtue for your own self, instead of using healthy food and exercise as a medium to becoming "'ripped and jacked" to fit within a certain ideal given for all. To strive for the latter result would be against the point of *The Stoic Body*.

Having the philosophical attitude of eating and exercising to live will naturally balance you out to your normal set point and how *you* are meant to be healthy. This is what I whole-heartedly believe to be the best option. This is the power of having a philosophical approach which correctly aligns the complexity of all this scientific detail and research through one simple ideology of doing something with variables that are under your control. Philosophy simplifies the complexity of it all. The important thing to remember is that for most people a proper diet and exercise programme will regulate the profile of the variables to your individual set point – it just takes time. Yes, it may sound pessimistic that we are all intrinsically born with a certain point that is programmed in us. This may frustrate you and dampen your motivation; but I don't see the merit in reacting like this. The purpose is to be healthy so that you have time for what truly matters – your intellect.

Returning to the set point theory, it would seem that undertaking a weight-loss programme in an attempt to revert the uncontrollable and tireless opponent of the set point is a waste. Research has shown us that when someone drops 10 per cent of their weight their metabolic rate can drop roughly 15 per cent in order to compensate. In this case exercise is very important, as fewer calories are burned everyday unless caloric expenditure is compensated through exercise.

Some researchers have claimed that exercise as well as certain anti-obesity medication can lower the set point in the sense that you provide a more favourable environment for your own ideal. The point is to add muscle. Muscle is metabolically active tissue. This means your BMR is increased proportionately to the quantity of muscle you have on your frame. The more muscle you have, the more calories you'll burn (greater thermic effect) by doing *nothing*.

BECOMING INTIMATE WITH POVERTY

> "Let us become intimate with poverty, so that fortune may not catch us off our guard. We shall be rich with all the more comfort, if we once learn how far poverty is from being a burden."
>
> – Seneca

PERIODIC CALORIC RESTRICTION

Fasting is a practice that was commonly used in the ancient world. Hippocrates, an ancient Greek physician, tells us: "Our medicine should be our food. But to eat when you are sick is to feed your sickness." Plato tells us that he fasted for improved physical and cognitive efficiency; his pupil Aristotle did the same.

Physical discomfort is something that we should embrace, and fasting is the perfect practice to start with. Understand that fasting was not founded by anyone, as nobody can claim something that we can all experience naturally. But the voluntary restriction of food is found in various religious and cultural traditions throughout history. We see this practice in Christianity, Judaism and most notably today during in Islam. During the month of Ramadan, Muslims around the world refrain from food, drink, sex, smoking and even anger from sunrise to sunset. Christianity, which came to power after the fall of Rome, held the belief that God is providence and abstaining from food pulls one closer to God. Seneca tells us: "Until we have begun to go without them, we fail to realize how unnecessary many things are."

This idea of being pulled closer to God was based on the fact that the suffering of hunger pains allows you to become more pure; when more pure, prayers are more likely to be answered. Becoming closer to ourselves – or in the context of religion, God – is becoming closer to the rational self. To the Stoics, living in accordance to nature is the deeper expression of every action they undertake. Fasting is a practice which is both frequent and necessary. It provides us with the perfect opportunity to allow ourselves to become closer to the rational self – and therefore more free, in a world where attachment to food has given us great trouble.

An interesting study looked at the eating habits of 28,000 children and 36,000 adults over the last thirty years. The results showed that the average time spent without food has decreased by one hour. Whether this is attributed to a sedentary lifestyle or not, I'm not sure, but I assume this is an important variable in the change which has come with the convenience of fast food. Fasting itself is still seen as eccentric, but this dubious attitude is changing. In recent years fasting has become the hot topic of scientific research. Increasingly, research has suggested that regular fasting is a way of *improving* health, rather than simply being a spiritual practice.

To some, the idea of fasting simply means to not eat; and while the practice of fasting involves abstinence from food it is *not* starvation. Since the idea of fasting is to restrict food, this can come across as very restrictive and invasive, and to some may give off the impression of an underlying problem with food. A poor relationship with food is exactly the opposite of what fasting aims to provide an individual with. A person who is starving has *no choice* whether they eat or not. Fasting is voluntary and temporary.

Research conducted at the Salk Institute for Biological Studies compared two groups of mice that were given both a high-fat diet and an equal amount of food. The only difference was that group one could eat whenever they pleased while group two were fasted for sixteen hours and fed for eight hours. The study lasted for 100 days and the results showed very clear differences between both groups. Mice which involuntarily fasted had put on 28 per cent less weight and showed signs of less liver damage, even though both groups had the same quantity of food available. Lower chronic inflammation in the fasting group suggests that overall this group of mice had reduced risks of encountering diseases such as stroke, Alzheimer's disease, heart disease and even cancer.

Studies over various species have shown an increased lifespan from caloric restriction. A study shows us that moderate caloric restriction increases the chance of survival in primate species, specifically in rhesus monkeys. Due to the similarities between rhesus monkeys and humans, the chance of human beings gaining the same benefits is likely, although not guaranteed. This is supported by many studies looking at caloric restriction in humans, which have shown significant improvement in their cardiovascular health.

Here are some common myths about intermittent fasting:

- It causes hypoglycaemia.
- The body is deprived of nutrients.
- It causes muscle loss. (In fact the opposite is true; fasting has been shown to promote greater muscle *retention* compared to those on a regular eating frequency.)
- It causes uncontrollable and overwhelming hunger, resulting in overeating.
- We require a constant supply of glucose for our cognition.
- It leads to a decreased BMR.

WOMEN AND FASTING

Most readers of this book are not female. I presume this based on the demographics of people attracted to Stoicism. However, it's important to briefly discuss the common concern of whether it's safe for women to intermittently fast. But first, let's quickly outline how the classical Stoics viewed gender, and whether this governs who can practise philosophy through fasting.

Musonius makes it clear that women as well as men have received reason from the gods. Women clearly have the capacity to judge between good or bad, what is right and what is wrong, and they too have the same senses as any man. He goes on to explain that both men and women have the capacity and the intrinsic inclination to move towards good. The same education and training is thus required for women. Stoicism is for both genders. If men and women are born with the same virtues, the same type of training and exercise is necessary.

Does this differ for fasting? The general consensus is that there are hormonal imbalances which occur in females in certain instances of caloric restriction. This isn't to say that a woman should never try fasting; it's just that if done incorrectly issues are possible. Women are very sensitive to signs of hunger. When the body is fasting, leptin and ghrelin are secreted in large amounts; the issue then becomes that hormone fluctuations are too extreme, which can lead to binge-eating, defeating the initial purpose of the fast.

For a woman, what is more appropriate (if fasting is to be undertaken) is to use the crescendo style, which is fasting two to three days per week, instead of every day. Some women will be able to do it every day, but not all. Generally crescendo is a good option as it will allow you to get the benefits of weight loss and cognitive enhancement, while avoiding the potential dangers of an everyday practice. With a crescendo style, you may choose two days of the week to fast, perhaps Wednesday and Friday, where on both days breakfast is missed and you eat between 12 p.m. and 8 p.m.

THE BREAKFAST MYTH

"Set aside a certain number of days, during which you shall be content with the scantiest and cheapest fare, with coarse and rough dress, saying to yourself the while: 'Is this the condition that I feared?'"

–Seneca

Imagine that there were no animals around for us to hunt, no fruit, no vegetables – no food at all. According to the logic of those opposed to fasting, we would become weak and incapable of functioning within a few hours. Does this seem realistic? In nature, food is not always abundant, so it makes sense that our bodies have become well adapted to provide us with the capability of hunting during periods of caloric scarcity. Does this means that since we have abundance our genetic nature changes? The answer is no. Our DNA doesn't comprehend what a supermarket is. The more I study the relationship between Stoic philosophy and its application to what is new in science, the more intriguing it becomes to see just how closely these ancient ideas align themselves to what the latest scientific research reveals.

So how does fasting exactly work? When should you do it? More importantly, why is fasting a better option than eating breakfast? Breakfast is a meal that we have come to respect as being the healthy and correct dietary decision. We've all heard these sayings: "Starting your day off right," and, "Breakfast is the most important meal of the day". Breakfast actually refers to the first meal of the day as "breaking your fast".

When you are in a fed state, this means that while your body is absorbing nutrients and storing energy as fat it is in the *postprandial* state. "Post" means "after" and "prandial" refers to food. When you are in a fasting state – after the body has completed the absorption of glucose and nutrients – your body enters what we call the *post-absorptive* state.

In a 2015 review of clinic trials (the largest to date – forty studies in total) from the journal of *Molecular and Cellular Endocrinology*, the effects of intermittent caloric restriction on frequent energy restriction overall resulted in "apparently equivalent outcomes" (body weight and composition). Fasting, however, had a more positive effect on reducing hunger.

Even if intermittent fasting makes no difference to weight loss, fasting has psychological benefits. An interesting study in 2011 from the Proceedings of the National Academy of Sciences looked at extraneous factors in judicial decisions. The study looked at judges' food breaks and decision sessions, comparing favourable rulings over time, respective to break frequency and duration. They concluded that as the day progresses, judges seem to lose their ability to make consistent rationally grounded decisions. However, there have been some critiques over this study because the result is more to do with specific cases. Regardless, the concept underlying the study, known as "decision fatigue", is very real. Decision fatigue is most often used as a phrase to understand the irrationality of impulse shoppers and impaired self-regulation. As the day progresses, judges become more inclined to make poor choices.

The same can be applied to the way we eat. Later in the day we crave more junk food. Many people snack late at night, ruining their caloric deficit during these late hours.

Intermittent fasting works well because it gives you leeway by restricting calories early on. You not only make better decisions from not suffering from decision fatigue, but you also give yourself an advantage by having so many calories abundant later on during the day. It's also easy to follow an hour-by-hour schedule instead of changing what you're eating in the sense of how many grams of carbohydrates. This all comes back to narratives, as with our previous discussion on the identity of certain dietary types. A vegetarian may find themselves consistent, disciplined and healthier as they follow their diet; the same with someone who follows a ketogenic diet or a vegan diet. We like to have rules; they serve us better in the long term rather than merely deciding to "eat healthier".

Diets such as veganism, vegetarianism or the ketogenic diet involve less decision making in the moment of "should I eat that?" This means less decision fatigue and more willpower.

Today it is very clear that there is a correlation between the foods we eat and the onset of oxidative and inflammatory stress (including very high levels of saturated fats and refined carbohydrates). High fibre and fruit do not cause oxidative stress and/or inflammation. Fat in the body, much like the food we consume, is a form of energy. This fat is stored in our body and acts as a physical lining for our organs in order to protect them from damage. Fat can also be fuel that is stored for when we are in need of energy and lack it elsewhere. From an evolutionary perspective we can observe this with animals intentionally gaining fat, or gathering food rich in fat, for the colder months of the year – for example, a squirrel gathering nuts. Humans are no exception to this system; it's our contemporary lifestyle which opposes the need for this sort of conservation.

If we use this same reasoning for intermittent fasting, but on a more micro scale, we see that the benefits work in much the same way. If you don't eat for a prolonged period of time, your body is going to inevitably gather energy from what it has internally stored, and this is a reason why many see caloric restriction as being symbolic of fat loss. This isn't to say that one can't gain weight fasting, but for most this would simply be nonsensical if gaining weight is a struggle in itself.

Insulin is produced in the pancreas and glucose comes from the carbohydrates we consume. Insulin is the driving force which converts carbohydrates into glucose and makes it readily available for us to utilise as fuel. Insulin's job is to stabilise blood sugar levels so that they do not rise too high (hyperglycaemia) or drop too low (hypoglycaemia). This energy is occasionally stored for future use when the input of energy is disproportionately large, and thus weight gain occurs. Insulin allows your body to use energy in future situations when required.

Once we eat food, especially a meal that is saturated with carbohydrates, our insulin levels increase significantly in order to help the body store energy. Glycogen is stored inside our liver through being linked into long chains (these peptide chains are also referred to as the A and B chain). In the liver, storage available is limited, and once the storage limit is reached the excess glucose is converted into fat through a process known as *de novo lipogenesis* (DNL). These fatty acids then undergo the chemical reaction *esterification*, which turns them into storage triacylglycerols (TG) to provide us with energy at later times through via beta oxidation. All you need to know about esterification is that it causes the body to gain fat.

The danger is that there isn't a particular limit of excess fat that can be stored as esterification is exacerbated through a disproportionate input to output. Our programming hasn't accounted for the invention of fast food restaurants; a limit wasn't accounted for. It's quite ridiculous when you think about the situation we've manifested for ourselves. Our "fat storage space" has a limit, and once that limit is reached the fat is stored in our bodies long term. This is directly related to the readily available glycogen in the body.

When you are in a fasted state your insulin levels decrease. This results in the body using stored energy that has undergone esterification as energy when input has ceased. Glycogen, which is glucose stored within your muscles and liver, is used as energy when required. This is depleted while you are in a fasted state. When you train, this energy is used and thus exercise depletes this glycogen even further. Glycogen depletion then has the potential to increase insulin sensitivity even further. After you are done with your workout, your body is able to store glycogen more effectively because energy will be utilised quickly to aid in the recovery of tissue. If you are not in a fasted state and do not exercise off stored glycogen, then the body recognises that glycogen stores are completely full and there isn't a higher probability of them being stored as fat (given a deficit of energy).

Although it's possible to lose fat while eating all day, the problem is that, except when you're asleep, the body doesn't experience the appropriate balance hormonally between being both fed and fasted. We have as a society prevented ourselves from allowing nature's intended hormonal balance to occur through the dogmatic idea of "boosting your metabolism by eating small meals frequently". Many people fear carbohydrates, especially sugar. But this is a bad attitude to have; we must simply understand the purpose of carbohydrates and also which types are more beneficial. Instead, many people exclude them completely (although doing this through the ketogenic diet has its own benefits). Intermittent fasting allows people to have nutritional flexibility, but still give their body the opportunity to experience a much-needed decrease in insulin levels. People enjoy the simplicity of tracking hours rather than grams of carbohydrates, and this is why I think fasting on a psychologically level is effective.

Ketosis

The ketogenic diet is based on dropping your carbohydrate intake to nearly zero. It's called this because at a certain point of restricting carbohydrates the body goes into *ketosis*, or increased levels of ketone bodies in the system, produced by the liver. Ketosis, or a ketogenic state, is achieved by the restriction of carbohydrates to a maximum of 50 g, or 10 per cent (or as low as 5 per cent) of one's total energy, according to the *American Journal of Epidemiology* in 2012. Protein consumption is to be kept at a moderate quantity of 1.2–1.5 g per kilo, according to the *International Journal of Environmental Research and Public Health*. The liver converts the fat you eat into ketones. These "ketone bodies" (beta-hydroxybutyrate, acetoacetate, and acetone) in particular can cross the blood-brain barrier, but these ketones can potentially – and do – serve as the body's main source of energy, given time, as the body becomes "keto-adapted" to "nutritional ketosis."

A great analogy Dr Jason Fung gives for understanding how fat and carbohydrates work is to imagine them as a fridge/freezer. The fridge (carbohydrates) is easily accessible and contains food which you can eat at will. The freezer (fat) has more food in it, higher density of calories, but is hard to access (you must thaw food or walk to the basement). So why would the body ever burn and utilise fat if it has carbohydrates (fridge available)?

As ketogenic diets work on similar merits to intermittent fasting, this can be a great alternative for females (as I previously mentioned), but also in combination with intermittent fasting which will provide a synergetic effect.

With today's reconstruction of Stoic doctrine comes the great influence of a pre-Socratic philosopher. Heraclitus believed in a similar concept to the Chinese philosophy of yin and yang. He told us that the universe works through the double interchangeable motion of opposing forces, which when in equilibrium is harmonic. On a biological level the importance of this harmonic exchange of polarities is very clear (night and day, hot and cold, life and death, order and chaos). It is the same for fasting, fed, insulin levels, essentially everything – but sleeping is not necessarily enough for this balance to occur.

As more research is released on nutritional ketosis and fasted ketosis and the potential alleviating effects for cognitive decline, the more I've coming to realise just how interlinked blood glucose is to willpower and motivation. Finding my sweet spot of blood sugar levels has been life changing.

FASTING THE RIGHT WAY

I've found intermittent fasting to work best by eating two large meals per day (without snacking.). By leveraging your sleep as part of your fast you can easily continue this throughout the morning, when appetite is naturally absent. Through an increase in caloric intake from morning to night, with the larger meal at the end of the day, we are able to work in sync with the body's natural shift of sympathetic "fight or flight" to the parasympathetic "rest and digest". Through *sympathetic* tone we have higher alertness, and we experience *parasympathetic* resting tone during the evening in a fed state as we relax. It's at this time we can eat our larger meals without having fatigue affect our productivity during our busy day.

I recommend the 16/8 schedule of fasting not because it necessarily produces better results physiologically, but because it is much easier to sustain for a longer period of time. This gradual transition to fasting reduces the chances the attempt will become a phase rather than a long-lasting habit. Sixteen hours fasted is simply skipping breakfast and then beginning your fed state at 12 p.m. and finishing at 8 p.m. There are other daily fasting regimes such as the Warrior Diet which consists of twenty hours fasted and four hours feeding. In this case you may fast until 4 p.m. and then finish feeding at 8 p.m. In saying that, if you are new to fasting, I strongly recommend starting with 16/8 to see how your body and mind react. Remember this is just an example, and you can adjust the times to suit your personal circumstances and schedule.

Daily fasting can be a very dramatic change. Following a more sporadic schedule can be a great way to either do it permanently (for women) or begin (for men). There are different ways to incorporate your first experiences of fasting into your life. The most straightforward and convenient way is fasting every time you travel or after a holiday celebration where you have eaten a lot of food. From successfully completing a 16-, 18- or even 24-hour fast you will realise that the human body is much more capable than we give it credit for. You may find yourself surprised by the lack of lethargy and hunger.

Dietary restriction is not only capable of increasing longevity, but evidence now suggests that alternative-day fasting or other forms of sporadic fasting can actually extend a person's lifespan. Alternative-day fasting is still a feasible method of fasting as fat oxidation increases, but studies have pointed out again and again that feelings of hunger don't decrease on the days where subjects are fasting, in comparison to the regular, everyday schedule. So, especially for men, sporadic and less frequent fasting will not be optimal if hunger is something you cannot "muscle through".

The protective outer lining of the stomach is more vulnerable during prolonged fasting periods and without frequent intake of food it can become more easily irritated. This calls for the gradual reintroduction of food after breaking a fast. Below you will find a list of food products ranked from best to worst (1-7) for the transition of fasting to feeding.

- Fruit and juices
- Vegetables
- Yoghurt (cultured)
- Grains and beans
- Dairy (non-cultured)
- Meat
- Processed foods

In a fasted state the body experiences several biological changes such as the production of enzymes in the digestive tract. Your digestive system needs time to adjust and reproduce the quantity of these enzymes. This reproduction is especially important when starting intermittent fasting or trying a more prolonged fast for the first time. Be sure to *slowly* reintroduce foods and use the list as a guideline from best to worst. Avoid anything that may irritate the stomach, including spicy and heavy foods. As this is a subjective thing, here's some advice.

Raw fruit is the best way to break a fast, as it's very light and easy on the system. However, avoid very acidic fruit juices (orange, lime, grapefruit) as too much will irritate your stomach. Aim to form a habit where after you break your fast, you move from lighter meals to heavier meals, smaller meals to larger meals, frequent meals to less frequent meals, etc. Find a way to progress in your food intake after breaking your fast. Foods you should avoid for breaking your fast are:

- Garlic
- Coffee
- Peppers
- Onion
- Soda
- Ginger

This isn't to say that you should refrain from enjoying a cup of coffee when fasted, as this has benefits of its own. Just don't overdo it. See how *your* body reacts. Although some may argue that you should have your biggest meal after your fasting period, this doesn't mean you should eat as much as possible right away. Eat a little fruit and see how your stomach reacts; from here gauge what you can handle. Over time you will find what works for you.

COGNITIVE PERFORMANCE AND DISEASE

The body becomes stressed when blood glucose levels increase. It's a stress that every part of the body experiences, including the brain. This stress on the brain is compensated for through brain-derived neurotrophic factor (BDNF). BDNF is a protein encoded by the BDNF gene and directly affects neurons belonging to the central nervous system and also the peripheral nervous system. BDNF supports the survival and growth of new neurons and synaptic pathways, which are key to sustaining long-term memory. Research from the *Proceedings of the National Academy of Sciences* in 2003 supports the link between BDNF and depression. However, only recently have researchers entertained the idea that lower BDNF levels may be a direct prognostic of the disease.

The hippocampus is the area of the brain where depression forms. Since fasting increases BDNF levels and antidepressants work on increasing BDNF levels, fasting may help to ameliorate symptoms of depression.. Whether this is conclusive or not, depressive states are very difficult to cure completely as many believe depression is a product of biological determinism. To anyone sceptical or even opposed to using fasting as a tool to combat this illness, my question to you is…why not? Why not try a practice which has many conclusive benefits of its own and may also help to improve a chronic ailment which for many is debilitating and often seems incurable?

Findings from the *Journal of Neuroscience Research* in 2008 found that fasting acts as neuroprotection for traumatic brain injury. Fasting isn't a miracle for the brain, but it can be used as an effective tool to reduce physical trauma. The brain doesn't suddenly protect you from trauma during times when you restrict food; rather, the brain has the ability to reduce oxidative stress, mitochondrial dysfunction and cognitive decline. Researchers used a controlled cortical impact (CCI) on rats who were in a fasted state. The CCI was developed around thirty years ago, using a testing platform in order to determine various biochemical properties of tissue in the brain when exposed to deformations. The research found that the rats who were under a twenty-four-hour fast, but not a forty-eight-hour fast, had brains with neuroprotective qualities.

We can see these neuroprotective qualities in a sporting scenario when an individual experiences a concussion after a heavy impact to the skull. It's not uncommon for a person in this situation to experience an instantaneous reduction of the appetite. I suspect this is evidence of neuroprotective adaptation of the body found by intentionally restricting calories. Research from the Committee on Nutrition, Trauma, and the Brain in 2011 looked at ketogenic diets as a way to reduce brain injury for military personnel and found a similar neuroprotective quality as with the 2008 findings. The committee suggested that the underlying mechanism involves ketosis rather than hypoglycaemia. Future research will be needed, but perhaps this means that ketogenic diets are much more effective than exclusively fasting as neuroprotective diets.

Alzheimer's disease (AD) is a neurodegenerative disorder characterised by cognitive decline. This cognitive decline is associated with the neuropathological hallmarks amyloid beta. These two peptides are crucial components of 36-43 amino acids which are central to the amyloid plaques commonly found in those who are suffering from AD.

A 2007 study from the *Neurobiology of Disease* journal hypothesised that because ageing is a large risk factor for cognitive decline and a restriction of caloric intake can slow down ageing (through a 40 per cent caloric restriction), theoretically this may slow down the loss of cognitive acuity in the case and/or risk of AD. The study concluded that restriction of calories and intermittent fasting regimens do ameliorate the age-related cognitive declines through processes that may relate to these pathologies.

Autophagy is a natural process of the human body which literally means "self-eating". Autophagy is the body's way of cleansing itself of waste, disease and other cells which are obsolete. These metabolic wastes are then used as molecules for energy to create new cells in the body. Colin Champ, M.D, assistant professor at the University of Pittsburgh Medical Center, put it this way: "Think of it as our body's innate recycling programme." Autophagy has also been shown to have a role in preventing inflammation and boosting immunity. In multiple studies rats have been genetically engineered to be incapable of the processing of autophagy. This was done to see exactly how important the process is for the regulation of the body. All subjects gained weight. They showed clear signs of increased fatigue and even slept more. They had higher cholesterol levels and impaired cognitive function.

Short-term fasting increases our ability to utilise autophagy; in theory this would then prevent various negative side effects occurring. Although some of these and multiple other studies are more conclusive than others, there is so much research being done with results being significant enough to further elaborate. They show that the relationship between fasting and autophagy is far from coincidental.

THE LOW-DOWN ON ARTIFICIAL SWEETENERS

Is it appropriate to drink zero calorie drinks when in a fasted state? There are a number of controversies around artificial sweeteners. Some claim they have cancerous properties; others say they make you fat. Those in the fasting world of health say that artificial sweeteners may spike insulin levels, thus ruining the purpose of fasting to lower insulin levels.

So what's the truth?

The American Heart Association and the American Diabetes Association agree that artificial sweeteners may be a viable option to combat obesity. The Food and Drug Administration (FDA) has approved the following sweeteners: stevia (low calorie), aspartame, neotame, acesulfame potassium (or acesulfame K), saccharin and sucralose. When you know a drink has zero calories, yet still tastes delicious – why wouldn't you try it?

Aspartame is a very common artificial sweetener found in various soft drinks and food. It has been around since 1965. A study in 1991 from the *Pharmacology & Toxicology* journal compared the effect of protein and aspartame. It found that protein produced an insulin response, while aspartame didn't. The same comparison was made in a 1990 study from *Metabolism* journal which compared insulin response with or without the combination of carbohydrates. Another study from *The American Journal of Clinical Nutrition* in 1989 showed that aspartame and its constituent amino acids had no effect on cortisol, prolactin, glucose and growth hormone. So it's pretty clear that aspartame does not have any direct effect on insulin levels.

An interesting study from the *Cellular Signalling* journal in 1998 isolated pancreatic cells and concluded that artificial sweeteners with a bitter aftertaste (acesulfame K, saccharin, stevia, and cyclamate – but not aspartame) were responsible for eliciting an insulin response when glucose is present. However, when fasted, glucose levels are somewhat drained.

Sucralose (also known as Splenda) uses dextrose as a bulking agent. Dextrose is a form of sugar, essentially glucose, and without a doubt it elicits a large insulin response. Sucralose activates receptors of sweetness in the taste buds. Some evidence points towards incretin hormones (which precede the secretion of insulin) being active through the response of receptive enteroendocrine cells in the gut. A 2010 review from the *British Journal of Nutrition* shows that in vivo studies (studies concerning the living) conclude that low-energy sweeteners such as sucralose or aspartame don't have effects on insulin, appetite or blood glucose, which was predicted by in vitro studies (performed with microorganisms, cells outside the normality of their biological context).

Research seems to show the insulin response to most artificial sweeteners is non-existent, but there are plenty of good reasons to avoid regular or even sporadic consumption. Disturbances of gut flora, the psychological dependency on sweets and concerns around long-term safety of prolonged consumption are the main caveats research has brought to light. Artificial sweeteners may prevent us from correctly associating sweetness to caloric intake; the negative conse-quence being that we willingly choose sweet foods elsewhere over those more wholesome and nutritious.

The most cited example is the San Antonio Heart Study where participants drank over twenty-one diet drinks every week and became twice as likely to be either overweight or obese in contrast to those who completely abstain. These are extreme quantities at first glance, but remember three per day (twenty-one per week) isn't unrealistic for many people today. In vivo studies suggest that the drinks are *very* addictive. Although short-term weight gain may not be a result of drinking these beverages, long-term consumption may exacerbate the harm of other nutritional choices in a person's diet, and this increases the likelihood of obesity in the long term. A 2007 study published in the *Public Library of Science* gave rats the choice between intravenous cocaine or saccharin (an artificial sweetener around 300-400 times sweeter than sucrose). The majority chose saccharin. It would appear that intense sweetness actually surpasses the cocaine reward.

Anyone remotely interested in overall health has heard time and time again about the importance of overall gut health (flora) for our overall well-being. According to 2010 research from *Microbe Magazine*, estimates for the number of human cells in the body stand at 37.2 trillion. Furthermore, going by the original estimate of 100 trillion bacterial cells being correct, the ratio of foreign to human is around 3:1. Clearly this means that many processes in the human body are exclusive of our own cells; frightening, but also humbling at the same time when you think about it! Our ability to extract energy from food is made possible by microbiomes which live in the gut. We now know that artificial sweeteners enhance the ability and efficiency of these microbiomes to extract energy from food and turn it into fat. In other words, intake of these artificial sweeteners harbours an environment more conducive making more calories available to us, according to Peter Turnbaugh from the University of California, San Francisco's biomedical sciences department.

Dr Christopher Gardner, an associate professor of medicine at Stanford University in California, when asked about artificial sweeteners, said: "While they are not magic bullets, smart use of non-nutritive sweeteners could help you reduce added sugars in your diet, therefore lowering the number of calories you eat. Reducing calories could help you maintain a healthy body weight, and thereby lower your risk of heart disease and diabetes."

There is some convincing evidence from the San Antonio Heart Study that artificial sweeteners can be addictive and cause weight gain over a seven- to eight-year period. In addition, various studies have shown a significant increased chance of metabolic syndrome (MS). Findings from the *American Journal of Clinical Nutrition* in 2012 show that the risk of developing type 2 diabetes more than doubled for participants in the highest quartile of diet beverage consumption, when contrasted to the controlled non-consumers. Within given age groups, the risk for coronary heart disease was significantly elevated in women who consumed more than two sweetened beverages per day, whether they contained sugar or artificial sweeteners.

Taken together, findings from all the studies suggest that consuming artificial sweeteners can be just as bad as normal sugar but *may* be an option worthy of consideration to reduce sugar consumption if used with strategy and detachment in mind. By no means am I advocating for you to drink these beverages on a daily basis – but drinking a Pepsi Max will not ruin your fasting experience.

Various functions of the gastrointestinal track are closely linked to our circadian sleep-wake rhythms. A simple example is blood flow increasing during the day; thus the metabolic responses to glucose are more gradual and slow during the night, as we are not nocturnal. According to a 2010 study from *Obesity Reviews* a disturbed circadian rhythm profile can affect gastrointestinal function and impair your metabolism and health. Wide empirical evidence supports the notion that fasting directly affects gut microbiota. The *Journal of Clinical Investigation* in 2011 concluded that the complexity of microbial life is very clearly correlated to obesity and metabolic dysfunction, giving an obese body a greater likelihood of gaining more energy through "obese microbiota" from food than "lean microbiota". This leads to overall changes in net input of energy, net expenditure and overall fat storage for different bodies.

How About a Cup of Joe?

Studies from New York, Columbia and Rockefeller universities have identified cells in the stomach which are responsible for animals' desire for food, even if they are not hungry. Rae Silver, head of the Laboratory of Neurobiology and Behaviour at Columbia University, and Donald W. Pfaff found a startling correlation between the release of a hormone called ghrelin and our ability to control our appetite.

Ghrelin is commonly referred to as the "hunger hormone". It is a peptide hormone produced by ghrelinergic cells in the gastrointestinal tract. Often only recognised as controlling and regulating our appetite, ghrelin also plays an important role in the delegation and regulation of energy throughout the body. As the stomach is stretched through satiation, secretion of ghrelin decreases rapidly. When the stomach is empty, the secretion of ghrelin increases. Hypothalamic cells in the brain increase our desire to eat food, and prepare the body for incoming food.

All animals have a circadian clock. This clock can be described as a subconscious rhythm of time that we work with. This schedule of time constitutes certain daily behaviours we have on the basis of hormone release. An example could be the large release of cortisol at 6 a.m., contributing to wakefulness; another example is the body reaching its lowest core temperature at 4 a.m. Ghrelin acts upon your habitual eating patterns, not an external factor set at a specific time. Your personal time-based decisions to eat food dictate the lessening or increasing rate of ghrelin secretion, rather than some sort of innate external driver such as the rise of the sun. This is fascinating and truly challenges the dogmatic belief that we require breakfast.

The collaborative study mentioned above shows that the

release of the hormone increases the appetite of rats, even when on a psychological level they are not feeling inclined to eat food. This results in the rats looking for something to eat in a frantic state. I briefly touched earlier on the phenomenon of smell causing a chain-like behavioural momentum of eating when we are not even hungry. According to a 2011 study from the *Journal of Neuroscience*, ghrelin enhances one's olfactory sensitivity and exploratory "sniffing" in both rodents and humans. The reports from the study showed that ghrelin increases the sensitivity to smell by decreasing the levels of odours around and enhances the probability of detecting, recognising and selecting food appealing to the individual. Since we're on the topic of smell, I'll mention this new 2017 study out of the University of California, Berkeley. This study actually suggests (based on rats) that our metabolism is tightly linked with our smell. Rats who lost their sense of smell lost more weight than rats who had their olfactory organs intact. All variables, such as caloric consumption and activity level, were controlled for. I should also mention that stem cells were left intact, meaning that they would regain their sense of smell after three weeks or so.

The power of ghrelin seems to be significant to the point where if high enough it can be extremely difficult to resist the urge to eat when your stomach is "thinking" for you. Perhaps this is where the phrase "don't think with your stomach" originates from. Ghrelin, which is released from cells in the stomach, travels through the bloodstream and into the brain, hindering our ability to make more grounded and rational decisions. There are plenty of circumstances where humans have been injected with ghrelin and their hunger has become noticeably higher, despite feeling full or satisfied before the injection.

Most of the hunger that you experience when you're fasting is simply your body not yet aligning itself to this schedule of eating. Your body *will* adjust, believe me. This will become much easier to overcome over time – take it as a personal challenge. Trust in the logic behind your body being able to adapt to a behaviour which is not ingrained in some sort of intrinsic schedule.

For some, simply understanding that this will take some time is not enough to help them make it through early stages of discomfort. Fortunately, there are other measures you can take to aid you in reducing your initial increase in appetite. If you are a coffee drinker, here is some great news: there is a direct relationship between appetite regulation and coffee consumption. Several empirical studies have shown that coffee may help overall weight loss. Caffeine specifically has often been used as an appetite suppressor; however it may not be the ideal beverage for this particular cause. A 2012 study from the *Journal of the American College of Nutrition* looked at whether the hormone peptide YY (PYY) is released more when coffee is consumed and whether this affects participants' hunger. PYY is produced in the gut and it gives us the feeling of being full in response to eating food – and it's interesting to note that obese people secrete far less PYY than people of a healthy weight. The study used four drinks, one being placebo-controlled. Subjects in the test had no idea what they were drinking. The three drinks were:

1. Caffeinated coffee
2. Caffeine-water solution
3. Decaffeinated coffee

More PYY simply means less hunger experienced. Levels of PYY decrease rapidly in the body after ninety minutes, but what was noteworthy is that the lessened hunger lasted for 180 minutes after ingestion; the increase of PYY also transcended through the consumption of glucose. Decaffeinated coffee was shown to have the largest appetite suppressing properties *by far*, and caffeinated coffee came in second place. Perhaps cholorgenic acid, or our hormones which promote satiety, are responsible for this. This is hard to understand for researchers as even the two hormones, ghrelin and leptin, which are strongly related to hunger, are ineffective on digestion. This doesn't mean that you have to drink more coffee, because this has risks in itself.

If you are a coffee drinker, sit down and think about how you can regulate your coffee fix to work in sync with the times during where you may be most vulnerable to cravings. It's interesting to occasionally switch your normal coffee for decaffeinated coffee. I did, and the effects on hunger were noticeable, even accounting for the anticipation and high expectations of it working. In theory, with this switch you can avoid possible attachment to caffeine too.

Coffee comes from roasting the seed from the *Coffea* plant's berries. The legend is that an Ethiopian goatherd actually found the magic of coffee while he watched his goats become super excited after chewing on these beans! It's interesting to note that a Harvard study published in 2015 by *Circulation* found that moderate coffee drinking is associated with a lower risk of an early death. Researchers evaluated the questionnaires from over 208,000 men and woman over thirty years of age. The research found that in comparison to those who don't drink coffee, those who drink on average between three to five cups of caffeinated or decaffeinated coffee, showed less risk of type 2 diabetes, cardiovascular disease, other neurological diseases such as Parkinson's and even suicide; which is astonishing. They believe that this is due to properties in coffee such as cholorgenic acid which is known to help reduce insulin resistance and inflammation, two variables associated with early onset of disease. However, there are many variables this study doesn't take into account, and therefore it can be dangerous to claim that "coffee is great for you". Coffee affects, not necessarily the length of sleep, but the quality, essentially disturbing the appropriate ratio of REM/NREM sleep – rapid eye movement versus non-rapid eye movement.

Coffee can also increase your stress and anxiety. Some of the wakeful effects that come from drinking coffee also produce a cortisol response via the adrenal gland. Research from Johns Hopkins Medical School show that the cognitive and mood benefits associated with caffeine intake are experienced because of the short-term reversal of caffeine withdrawal. Researchers found that cognitive performance was not increased when there was no caffeine withdrawal. The only way to get back to baseline is to drink coffee again, and this is where the dependant danger emerges, a danger which can cancel out any benefits previously mentioned. As with any stimulant, caffeine is physiologically and psychologically addictive. Because blood pressure increases, shallow breathing occurs and the brain is deprived of oxygen. This handicap on your rational and calm thinking can affect your emotional intelligence (EQ). Also don't forget the risk coffee poses to your sleep. If you drink coffee at 9 a.m., 25 per cent of it will still be in your body at 9 p.m. This is why it is common advice (and rightly so) to restrict caffeine consumption to the morning hours.

Use it when needed, at the appropriate times, whether to improve your experience in a fasted state, help regulate your appetite or perform better during exercise. Don't make the mistake of becoming attached to coffee to perform what you should be able to do without it.

Constantly test your attachment to something, because you may not realise you are attached until you are extremely attached. Remember that the mind is great at rationalising the irrational and frequently blinds you. If you insist on drinking coffee, then flip a coin twice every morning. If it lands on tails twice then you can have your two coffees; twice on heads, no coffee (just tea); one of each, then you can drink one cup. A practice like this will very quickly expose any attachments and dispositions/tendencies you may have.

The World Health Organisation concluded that coffee should no longer be considered a carcinogen, although drinking very hot coffee can increase the risk of cancer. According to the analysis, drinking very hot beverages is one probable cause of oesophageal cancer and that it is the temperature, rather than the drinks themselves, that appears to be responsible. Coffee consumption may well have positive effects for the liver as well as helping prevent uterine cancers. This will no doubt be a relief to the well over 50 per cent of people in developed countries who drink coffee (some reports claim 84 per cent of adults in the United States are regular drinkers). Well over twenty years ago the *New England Journal of Medicine* told us that drinking two cups of coffee per day increased the risk of pancreatic cancer by 2.1 times – and closer to 3 times for those who drink five cups per day. Several years later, research concluded that there was actually no correlation between pancreatic cancer and coffee.

Coffee is the classical example of the complexity of modern health literature today. One day it's healthy, the next it's deadly. This is the same with red wine, or chocolate – today's poison is tomorrow's medicine. Through the years it was speculated that regular coffee increased cholesterol, so people then switched to decaf. But then it was found out that harmful industrial solvents were used to exclude caffeine to create decaf. I could go on for hours covering the opposing literature on the topic, back and forth between study and study, but my answer will still be the same. Take the popularised words of Aristotle into consideration: "All things in moderation."

"There is no reason, however, why you should think that you are doing anything great; for you will merely be doing what many thousands of slaves and many thousands of poor men are doing every day. But you may credit yourself with this item – that you will not be doing it under compulsion, and that it will be as easy for you to endure it permanently as to make the experiment from time to time...We shall be rich with all the more comfort, if we once learn how far poverty is from being a burden."

– Seneca

As with any other Stoic practice involving the physical self, there needs to be a clear distinction made between voluntary discomfort and masochism. You must not believe that the merits of fasting don't come with consequences if abused through expectations of greater achievement – this is foolish. What is also important to disclose to yourself for your own ego is that you are not doing anything special by simply adhering to how your body is *meant* to function. To contemplate, even for a brief moment, that you are going to forgo frequent eating out of selfish convenience is an act that Seneca would have been sure to denounce. There is no reason you should think you are doing anything great, as you simply are following in the footsteps of slaves who came before you. The first step is to understand that you're not going to die from going a few hours without food. By approaching your first time fasting as something which is going to be uncomfortable is undoubtedly going to lead to failure. I believe it's not worth attempting to live a lifestyle that doesn't have the potential for longevity in the first place.

Intermittent fasting will not be ideal for everyone in the long term as a daily practice for various reasons (gender, social or logistical). What I *am* adamant about is that everyone should intentionally fast throughout various periods of their lives to essentially rehearse poverty. We must all at some point reaffirm gratification if the opportunity is given – which it is, every single day of every single hour. Fasting is a perfect embodiment of one of the key virtues of Stoic philosophy and it is manifested in a practice that as a by-product opposes one of our greatest challenges as a society: obesity. Allow fasting to *allow you* to appreciate the abundance of food you have available to you. Resist the temptation of vice and gluttony that comes with the delusion that the availability of food is something you have undoubted control over. The likelihood of food becoming scarce lessens the more fat we seem to get; the fatter we get, the more we believe food *is* in our control, and thus the more of a problem it has become.

PART FOUR:
PROOF OF PROGRESS

"Since a human being happens to be neither soul alone nor body alone, but a composite of these two things, someone in training must pay attention to both. He should rightly pay more attention to the better part, namely the soul, but he should also take care of the other parts, or part of him will become defective. The philosopher's body also must be well prepared for work because often virtues use it as a necessary tool for the activities of life."

– Musonius Rufus

PHYSICAL TRAINING

The Stoic does not prioritise physical training, but recognises the merit in its potential to aid the evolution of the soul. Musonius explains to us the importance of intentionally enduring discomforts such as cold and heat. Seneca swam in cold waters instead of bathing for the usual purpose of social discourse. This doesn't necessarily exclude more common athletic training, such as strength training, being a viable option today.

However, Epictetus decries intense and repeated training of the body as an act which is anything but virtuous. To him, the obsession of the naked philosopher who disregards the body and rejects the importance of it is a more valuable commodity to have than the athlete who is obsessed with training it. It is not the physical training itself Epictetus is against, but the reasoning behind the act. (It could be because Epictetus had a disabled leg, and some stories say it was broken by his master. He was not an athletic man by any means.)

Epictetus does provide us with a fascinating insight into the suggested methodology of physical training a Stoic today would follow. In his *Discourses* we come to understand that Stoics believe progress in philosophy is not determined by how many books you have read, or even how many books you have written. Progress to the Stoic is determined by the outcome, or the proof of progress. The results and the true visible changes that come to existence in your life – this is the proof. This is not an argument to claim that progress must be external in a physical sense; simply that something must be observable by the external for it to be recognised.

Epictetus claims that to see someone's philosophy on physical training you must look at that person's shoulders. Instead, most look at the equipment they use or the frequency they train. Epictetus says: "Suppose, for example, that in talking to an athlete, I said, 'Show me your shoulders,' and then he answered, 'Look at my jumping weights.' Go to, you and your jumping weights! What I want to see is the effect of the jumping weights." Talk is cheap. It is easy to exaggerate about what you *claim* to have the capacity to do in a future situation; or more comically, what you *plan to do* when your circumstances are "just right". In an era where most understand the merit of health, there's too much emphasis on what's new, what works and, as Epictetus phrases it, "look at my jumping weights".

This is an egotistical display and lacks genuine self-examination of what truly warrants celebration.

I think everyone must achieve a solid base of strength for three reasons:

- Strength is quantifiable and progress is somewhat linear and structured.
- Strength training reveals your weaknesses.
- Strength is a transferable athletic aptitude.

Some people will argue that it's important to choose one aspect of fitness/sport and excel in it, and while I do agree that this is something everyone can do, it's just not a viable option for beginners. Think of strength training like school. You learn how to use your mind, discovering your strengths and weaknesses, and after you graduate school you move onto the esoteric endeavours. In this case think of graduating school as achieving a fundamental base of strength.

Now this isn't to say that cardio is bad; if you hate weight training then by all means, swim, run and jump. If we compare the advantages and disadvantages of buying a house versus renting, in most cases buying a house is the better option if you have the means to pay off the mortgage. This money ends up in asset you own, while rent is simply throwing money away in exchange for a living space. You maintain the ability to use the money or the asset of the purchased home (if there is no major economic crash or lack of income). Likewise we keep muscle as an asset to burn off calories passively.

Author Stephen Covey once said that an individual who spends hours a day running has probably gained many years in their life due to the running, but all these extra years were probably spent running (ha!). It should also be noted that within "building muscle" is sprinting, otherwise known as high intensity interval training (HIIT). HIIT seems to be treated as a recent and trending discovery, but Seneca advised us on a similar idea: "Now there are short and simple exercises which tire the body rapidly, and so save our time; and time is something of which we ought to keep strict account. These exercises are running, brandishing weights, and jumping…But whatever you do, come back quickly from body to mind."

Don't be fooled into thinking there is anything particularly special about HIIT. A 2017 systematic review and meta-analysis by *Obesity Reviews* showed us that there is no advantage of interval training (HIIT) over moderate intensity continuous training on body fat. It's the use of time which is important here. The idea is that you want to put in the least amount of time and effort for the biggest results. This should not be mistaken with laziness; rather it is efficiency. According to Seneca, this will create worthy shoulders, not a light jog for hours on end. The idea is to burn calories, not time. Listen to a podcast or music while you run; or listen to nothing at all and instead focus on your breathing. For the best results for your overall well-being, combine yoga, weights, callisthenics, Qi Gong, running and basketball, and don't become compliant with only one form of exercise. The ancient Greeks when training for war would their entire body. This was a principle which ancient athletes swore by.

Athletic contests were an integral part of social and spiritual life in Greece. Many contests were held in honour of heroes and gods. The gymnasium became intimately connected with education as well as medicine. The Academy, the Cynosarges and the Lyceum are examples of the three main public gymnasia. The Cynosarges was a public gymnasium, which was where Antisthenes was said to have lectured.

Milo of Croton was a champion wrester from the city of Croton. He was said to carry a bull on his shoulders every day. As the bull grew bigger, this increased the weight he would have to carry and he grew in his strength. The same principle applies to any reasonable weight training programme and success, otherwise known as progressive overload. A programme called Stronglifts 5x5 is the most simple, easy to follow, effective and efficient programme, with only three workouts per week. Thousands of people around the world have used this programme because it *works*. There are a few workout programmes I think are good for beginners.

I'm not advocating for you to abstain from cardiovascular training or to say that it's obsolete. Aerobic exercise is still an integral part of my training today – more so than ever. Research from *Sports Medicine* in 2011 revealed that exercise is at least as good as the best antidepressant medications available. Exercise also allows the body to clear the bloodstream of something we call *tutor necrosis factor* (TNF). TNF is a pro-inflammatory signal which increases your sensitivity to pain and inhibits muscle growth, as well as increasing your risk of blood clot formation, according to a 2005 study by the journal of *Arthritis Research & Therapy*. I will tell anyone I am coaching to first build a base of muscle. Cardio can be included of course: twenty minutes per day of fast-paced walking or playing sport is the way I recommend you do this to supplement weight training.

Get into the habit of going to the gym at the same time, on the same days, for the same duration. Consistency will be key to your success or failure. Select a programme that suits your schedule, experience and ability; normalise it and *do not stop*. For most people, going to the gym is never going to be convenient. There's something else the majority of people would prefer to do. Never miss a day in the gym.

I'll leave you with this quote by Pierre Hadot: "The notion of philosophical exercises has its roots in the ideal of athleticism and in the habitual practice of physical culture typical of the gymnasia. Just as the athlete gave new strength and form to his body by means of repeated bodily exercises, so the philosopher developed his strength of soul by means of philosophical exercises, and transformed himself. Exercises of body and soul thus combined to shape the true person: free, strong and independent."

PRACTICAL POSTURE

Posture is simply defined as the way you hold your body upright while standing, while you lie on your bed or sit in a chair. Furthermore, "good" posture describes the alignment of your body in a way which allows supporting muscles, tendons and ligaments to be free of strain (including during any activity). Never in my life have I met a client who, on further assessment, didn't need at least some improvement in posture. Your posture should correct somewhat with a consistent training programme, but there are active measures you can take to improve more quickly and efficiently.

The way you hold your body is a solid representation of your internal state. Thus, if you are living with the philosophy to revoke morally bad reactions to the external world, it is a wise decision to recognise the importance of having a well-aligned body. The reaction to the external world is a form of strategy; this strategy is much harder to play well while your shoulders sag, your body is closed, your head falls towards the ground and your power and rigidity is made fragile.

Benefits of good posture:

- The alignment of your joints and bones are fixated correctly. Movement of your muscles are optimised.
- Reduced risk of arthritis as the likelihood of joint wear and tear is lessened.
- Less stress on all your ligaments, which hold your spine and joints in place.
- Improved confidence, the ability to speak clearly and pronounce your words.
- Lessened muscular aches and lower back pain
- Fatigue is lessened as your muscles are being used optimally.
- Overall appearance improves.
- A longer and healthier life. People who consistently have good posture are less likely to die from various

illnesses. A recent Australian study showed that after age twenty-five every hour of bad posture as a by-product of watching TV reduces a person's life expectancy by 21.8 minutes!

POSTURE AND SELF-AWARENESS

Choose a specific colour or object that you see frequently and attach the thought of good posture – or one or more of these following psychological cues – to it. Each time you see it act according to the relevant technique.

- Walk as if you are balancing an object on your head.

- Lift your chest up, retract your shoulder blades by lifting them up and then pulling them down and back. The distance between your hip bone to your rib cage should be noticeable.

- Level your chin. The highest point of your body is not the front of your head but the top region of the back. Practice this by relaxing the jaw, muscles in the neck and relaxing your upper lip.

- Stand with your feet shoulder width apart. Your legs should be at their longest point, but without being entirely locked. Keep the weight of your body on the balls of your feet. By doing this you prevent misalignment.

- While you are walking, bounce through your calves rather than simply stepping firmly on the ground.

- Pretend there is a straight line or a string that is going through your body from the top of your head, pulling you vertically.

- When beginning any strength training programme, do not let your ego get in the way of the needed repetition with light weights and good form, to reinforce good posture in the beginning stages.

- Be sure to always stretch following workout routines; this should be clarified in detail as you read into your programme of choice.

There are many free only resources to help you with posture. Using yoga to stretch out your chest, hamstrings and hips can make a big difference.

Our Adaptive Advantage

Evolution can be defined as the heritable components of a specific population's ability to change and adapt over successive generations. Charles Darwin proposed that the characteristics which make creatures better adapted to their surrounds will have a greater chance of survival and therefore reproduction. As time passes, these creatures will continue to adapt better properties, until the new evolved species has a mixture of the best possible character traits for survival.

Since the beginning of culture itself, man has always been curious about the origins of himself. Whether religion is the vehicle used to find this, or whether science is, the point still remains universal that we share an intrinsic curiosity about life's big questions. With our evolution comes various unique abilities which separate us from other species. What excludes us from the rest of animals? The ability to speak, to synthesise opposing ideas. The concept of Hegelian dialectic comes to mind as an appropriate description of our cognitive acuity – comprising a thesis, a reaction, an antithesis, contradicting the thesis and therefore creating tension, only able to be resolved through a synthesis. I think we can all agree this is a very human-like trait exclusive to our intelligence as a species.

Through the ages, as we evolved, we developed the ability to use complex tools. Most noteworthy of all, we began to stand upright or became bipedal (*biped* meaning "two feet", from Latin *bis* "double"; *pes* "foot"). Many scholars now agree that because we were able to walk on two feet, our hands became free and this freedom of physical manipulation and alteration of the world around us followed this exponential growth in intelligence which today excludes us from other animals. The evolutionary pressure which resulted in the freedom of our hands also came with the development of nerves and finely tuned muscles in the palm and fingers. According to the endurance running hypothesis bipedalism gave us a greater capacity to be self-aware through our enhanced field of vision; we are slower at first over short distances covered by foot, but over longer distances we are superior to other animals.

Most people will experience some sort of back pain throughout their lives (occasionally debilitating) and often this is not a result of any specific incident; rather it's the consequence of cumulative degeneration. This rightly raises the question of the integrity of our spine's design. Although it seems logical to attribute our backaches to our sedentary lifestyles, this is not necessarily the *only* reason. Perhaps this is an issue which is more out of our control than most perceive it to be. Carol Ward, an anthropologist and anatomist from the University of Missouri in Colombia tells us, "The problem is that the vertebral column was originally designed to act as an arch." What Dr Ward is saying is that as we became bipedal (in order to support the weight of our head and balance optimally over the hip and leg joints), the spine naturally curves to compensate for this weight. Because of this, lordosis of the lower back and kyphosis of the upper back is common. The S curve we naturally have in our backs is useful as it allows us to be more efficient with our energy. But with this comes pressure on the lower back in an upright stance – and even more so in a seated position.

The joints in our back are very delicate and complex. We are the only mammal that is able to lean back and arch the spine (hyperextension). With this ability comes more twisting and pivoting of the disks between the vertebrae. Movement in the lower back region is often felt to be painful and uncomfortable during heavy lifting. This isn't exclusive to lifting objects and being active – the way you sleep is also a common example of this discomfort in action.

"We've known for a long time, since Darwin's time, that humans have evolved, and that humans are not perfect, because evolution doesn't produce perfection," said Jeremy DeSilva, an anthropologist at Boston University. Bruce Latimer, a paleoanthropologist at Case Western Reserve University extends this idea by stating humans are the only mammals which can physically have scoliosis. Dr Latimer explains that *Homo erectus* (such as the Lucy skeleton from 1.5-3 million years ago) had lateral curvature in the spine – clearly not having a cell phone and a couch to lie on for hours on end.

The body simply compensated for this outstanding opportunity. Selection for bipedalism outweighed the issues that came with it. If we look at our genomes as verbalised thoughts, their internal dialogue would come across as something like this: "Bipedalism is going to be incredibly useful and anything negative that may result from this adaptation is not significant enough to prevent this adaptation from occurring." The clearest example is the ability to read this very sentence.

Clearly there are still many questions on why exactly we became bipedal and how exactly our unique intelligence came about. Perhaps these questions will never fully be answered. Some say it is exclusively for the ability to reach fruit or being able to travel long distances in order to reach it; others speculate that it's for our ability to scan the horizon for predators and prey. The *savannah theory* postulates that bipedal locomotion favoured the scarcity of food commodity due to the drying of African forests in the Miocene period.

There are other, more outlandish, theories for our intelligence. An example is the controversial *stoned ape theory*, postured by Terence McKenna. He argues that our intelligence came through the discovery and experimentation with psychedelic substances. Mr McKenna argues that the large gap and exponential growth of our cognitive ability coincides with the prevalence of psilocybin mushrooms through a specific period. What is very clear is that more work needs to be done to understand the factual origins of both our intelligence and reason for walking on two legs. A fascinating book to read on this topic is Daniel Lieberman's book: *The Story of the Human Body: Evolution, Health, and Disease.*

Our world today provides unfavourable circumstances for our already vulnerable spines. What is worse than simply being upright is to be sedentary for the majority of the day, as many of us often are. This act opposes and revokes our natural inclination to utilise our adaptive advantage and be in constant locomotion. If we became bipedal as an adaptive strategy and became more intelligent through freeing up our hands, does this mean that our modern lifestyle is lessening our intelligence? Perhaps this would explain the copious amount of memes on the internet. Of course I'm joking, but perhaps an evolutionary biologist reading this can entertain the thought (or laugh at me).

WALKING AS MEDITATION

When we stand up, various cellular functions involving cholesterol and blood sugar activate within ninety seconds of moving. When you are seated your blood flow is constricted which allows fatty acids to accumulate. Your metabolism slows and you burn fewer calories when you are seated. Your cardio-vascular system is affected.

When you are seated your abdominals are not being used; when you stand they are activated. If your abdominal muscles are inactive too often, coupled with a lack of direct isolation of the muscle, they may atrophy. This will weaken your core strength which will contribute to more back pain.

When you sit, your food isn't able to digest because your gastrointestinal tract is being compressed together. When this occurs there are various other side effects such as pain or cramping, constipation and general discomfort.

Your hips will inevitably become tight with hours spent sitting in a similar position.

Here are some practical methods for dealing with these issues:

- Set a vibrating alarm on repeat while you're working every thirty to sixty minutes. When it vibrates, stand up, move around and stretch.

- Create a standing workstation or focus on improving the ergonomics of your seated working area.

- Become more aware of the decisions you make during the day. For instance, walk up the stairs instead of taking the lift.

- Create an environment where you are forced to stand more often. Place frequently used objects slightly further away than you usually would. Get creative!

> "We should take wandering outdoor walks, so that the mind might be nourished and refreshed by the open air and deep breathing."
>
> – Seneca

No animal has trouble moving its body. All beings in the animal kingdom are dexterous with the use of their limbs. There is no confusion to an animal about how its body is meant to move, as this is a function which is instinctive from birth. There is no need to *think* and *contemplate* how to lessen the strain of their movement, as there is no external influence affecting their ability to live according to nature. Through the bustling and noisy streets of Athens, vendors would shout, the *agora* was lively, tradesmen were at work; every crevice of the city was filled with energy. Walking was an important activity for the philosopher. Walking would clear the mind and allow one to experience new insights through interacting with the physical world.

As Seneca explains, the act of wandering outdoors nourishes our minds not only through the external environment but through the power of open air and the irresistible urge to breathe in deeply. Nietzsche would later say: "It is only ideas gained from walking that have any worth."

- When you get stressed or overwhelmed, take a walk.
- When you have a tough problem to solve or a decision to make, take a walk.
- When you are tired and fatigued, take a walk.
- When you need some air, take a walk.
- When you have a phone call to make, take a walk.
- When you need exercise but lack energy, take a long walk.
- When you have a meeting or a friend over, take a walk together.
- Heck, walk while you read this book.

A simple walk will allow you to escape cyclical thoughts and provide you with a "clean slate", while also allowing your body to move in its natural locomotion. This will provide some balance with today's lifestyle. While you walk you will once again come to the realisation of how perfectly happy you can be right now.

PART FIVE:
BREAKING TENSION

"If you are distressed by anything external, the pain is not due to the thing itself, but to your estimate of it; and this you have the power to revoke at any moment."

– Marcus Aurelius

UNDERSTANDING CORTISOL

Cortisol is known as the "stress hormone", and it has very direct physiological effects on us. Cortisol is produced in the adrenal cortex. The output of cortisol is based on a myriad of reasons (mostly expected diurnal variation). This hormonal secretion aligns to specific times of the day – high in the morning and low in the evening. Cortisol is not stress itself, as it's commonly described. Cortisol is a hormone which *responds* to stresses such as depression, dependencies, various disorders, pregnancy and intense physical activity. All these are examples of individuals with excessive cortisol profiles. To quickly elaborate the point that stress itself isn't cortisol itself, think about a top-tier athlete. Their physical activity is the stress which the cortisol *responds* to after intense physical exertion.

One of the most important functions of cortisol is allocating energy for the body through the metabolisation of fat and carbohydrates. This metabolic process increases our insulin response. This response is responsible for changes in blood sugar levels. The increase or decrease of insulin and thus cortisol also has a significant effect on our appetite and physiological composition. In Palaeolithic times, cortisol was necessary to our survival, keeping us alert and reducing the need to sleep during periods where an individual or group may be prone to predation, invasion or any other stress-provoking situations (such as scarcity of food).

Although our world today is very different, cortisol is not obsolete as a hormone. The reason why it has become an issue frequently spoken about is because our environment does not a support a healthy amount of its release. In urban settlements cortisol is increasing rapidly year by year as we adopt a work-centric lifestyle. A 2013 study from the *International Journal of Environmental Research and Public Health* shows that higher levels of neighbourhood green space [parks and trees] in deprived urban communities are linked with lower perceived stress and a steeper diurnal decline in cortisol secretion.

The moment we bite into food – even before the food reaches the stomach – the incretin system is activated. Incretin is a hormone which comes from the specialised cells of the small intestines into the bloodstream. As you consume a meal your blood glucose levels rise and incretins then stimulate the production of insulin in the bloodstream as food matter breaks down. Insulin regulates the metabolisation of carbohydrates, fat and protein by providing the capability to absorb glucose from the blood. When this glucose is absorbed from the blood it can be stored as fat in our liver and also in other skeletal muscular cells. While we are fasted cortisol actually works on several different systems to increase the glucose available for later use.

If we compare cortisol and insulin they appear to have opposing functions. Cortisol prepares the body for wakefulness and action, while increased insulin allows the body to store energy and can quickly make us feel lethargic. Cortisol increases the blood sugar in our bodies, while insulin lowers it. As you know by now, increased insulin is correlated to an increased risk of obesity. If cortisol raises insulin, naturally insulin should decrease with a decrease in cortisol. A decrease in cortisol drives a decrease in insulin and then there's a lack of fat storage, furthermore a decreased risk of obesity.

Dr Jason Fung explored the correlation between cortisol and insulin using the example of Cushing's syndrome (CS). CS is a debilitating disorder where excessive cortisol production from both the adrenal and pituitary gland increases blood sugar and the risk for diabetes. What is fascinating about this disease is that the most visible consequence is weight gain (94 per cent of patients). The disease is associated with obesity as seen in subclinical cases, where glucose and insulin were elevated to a similar level. In population scenarios where CS is not the focused variable, cortisol rates are still correlated to BMI and overall waist measurements (as shown in a random sample taken in Glasgow, Scotland). This isn't by chance; the correlation between cortisol and weight is becoming increasingly more evident as we all become more stressed.

The correlation between weight and cortisol levels is clear with those who have higher saliva cortisol levels and people with urinary cortisol excretion. These individuals *all* have higher BMI and waist to hip ratios. Cortisol levels are controlled by a specific enzyme located in adipose (fat) tissue, which is responsible for converting inactive cortisone to active cortisone. Adipose tissue is formed through stored energy and used to cushion and protect the body. Fat which surrounds our stomach and intestines (visceral fat) has more of this enzyme inside it.

As I previously mentioned, 94 per cent of CS patients showed increased body weight, but interestingly 97 per cent had an increase of fat specifically in the abdominal area. Fat in this area has greater volumes of blood flowing to the relative size of the blood vessels. Coincidently roughly four times the amount of cortisol is readily available to access this area in contrast to subcutaneous fat, once again reinforcing just how connected cortisol is to local fat storage. Visceral fat cells are known to form densely in the gut area, enlarge and thus become symbolic of the caricatured belly of the diabetic and obese.

We can further validate this relationship by looking at the contrary consequence of insufficient cortisol levels. People with Addison's disease (AD) suffer from adrenal insufficiency. This entails a very low release of cortisol, with both cortisol and aldosterone often lacking in AD patients. As with CS, one of the most noticeable side effects is on weight – but patients with AD lose weight rather than gain it.

For the ordinary person, this is not as relevant, as AD and CS are both extreme examples. However, this is exactly Dr Fung's point – our so-called "normal" hormonal levels *are* excessive. This correlation to weight gain/loss from the changes in hormonal levels may perhaps be a wake-up call to how little we are paying attention to the significance of distress as a precursor to obesity, rather than completely isolating the issue to caloric intake. Cortisol is a factor which at a certain point is larger than and precedes the success of upholding a consistent caloric deficit. People say you are what you eat; one could also say you are what you think, to some extent.

THE PARADOX OF CORTISOL

Cortisol is found in various body fluids including urine, blood and saliva. From these samples there are various forms of cortisol which can be measured: cortisone (inactive), free cortisol (active), metabolites of cortisone and cortisol formed as a by-product of enzymatic activity. According to a 2009 study from *Progress in Neurobiology*, the mood dysfunction found in extreme cases of high cortisol (in this case CS) is likely attributed to the higher activation of glucocorticoid receptors which have specific intersections with 5HT1A (a subtype of the 5-HT receptor), binding to serotonin and norepinephrine. The idea is that cortisol levels on the surface can only tell us so much. Cortisol metabolism differs for individual enzymatic expression.

A 2008 study from *The Journal of Clinical Endocrinology and Metabolism* looked at seventeen obese men who were asked to eat to whenever they wished. Group one ate a high fat and low carbohydrate diet (66 per cent fat, 4 per cent carbohydrate – virtually the ketogenic diet) and group two ate a moderate carbohydrate diet (35 per cent fat, 35 per cent carbohydrate) for four weeks. The conclusion of the study was that for group one, blood cortisol increased, clearance decreased and due to an increase of 11β-HSD1 activation in the liver, regeneration increased. Ketogenic diets show that on the surface cortisol is increasing but the effect on reversing MS is positive, hence the appearance of a paradox. Group two lost a similar amount of weight but showed no change to their cortisol profiles (no effect in 11β-HSD1 activation).

Cortisol increases in ketogenic diets and prolonged fasting, which shows us that fat loss is still possible despite increased cortisol secretion (which makes sense, as a deficit is the key variable). Some of the seventeen obese men had high perceived stress and high fat but average or even below average levels of serum cortisol.

Fasting and ketogenic diets are almost like an exception to the rule. We could refer to them as a *eustress* (good stress) contrasted to a *distress* (bad stress). A eustress is good in the sense that it is later compensated for, despite being taxing in the moment.

However, if stress is a big problem for you in general, proceed with caution for fasting. Extended fasts or everyday fasts may not be the ideal option for you if you have a propensity for stress. As previously covered, always come back and consider the hierarchy of needs (calories → macronutrients → micronutrients → meal timing [fasting] → supplements). The sporadic schedule may be more appropriate plan for you if you are sensitive to stress. Instead of fasting you may take on the challenge of reducing sauces and spices, and eating more plain and simple food, focusing on the quality of food you are eating.

I believe the difference between females and males is closely related to our Palaeolithic gender roles (not to be mistaken as societal roles). Most evolutionary anthropologists have come to agree that the majority – some speculate upwards of 80 per cent – of food for tribal communities was supplied by women, while the men's hunting only supplied 20 per cent (these are estimates, but the general ratio is true). Males were/ are more tolerant to prolonged fasting (we could equate this to an everyday practice or a sporadic and prolonged fast) as small groups of men would follow large animals for longer periods of time while women gathered grains, various seeds, nuts, fruits, grubs, smaller animals and insects.

Interesting findings from a large survey by the *American Psychology Association* show that women are more likely than men (28 per cent versus 20 per cent) to report having a great deal of stress. Additionally women are more likely (31 per cent versus 21 per cent) to report that they eat as a coping mechanism in response to stress and again, women reported eating too much/unhealthy food in the previous month due to stress (49 per cent versus 30 per cent) at the time of the survey.

This is a supposition, but I see potential correlations being made between the ratio of overweight men to women – there are more men than women – being somewhat caused by the homogenised style of eating we all follow. Perhaps this style opposes the male's natural hunting instinct. It's also widely accepted that physiologically men are intended to live in leaner physiques. Of course it doesn't make sense to simply blame this one possibility. I think it's clear that the increase in obesity is caused by a myriad of variables. The homogenisation of eating styles is one possibility; our increasingly sedentary nature is another (rather obvious); but also something as seemingly unrelated as war and military conscription.

Dr Robert Sapolsky from Stanford University explains that there are no consistent differences in cortisol production between genders. Dr Sapolsky argues the hormone oxytocin, more abundant in females, could be the dividing variable responsible for perceived stress in females opposing the very outdated and dogmatic idea that males and females have distinct differences in cortisol secretion. What I propose is that ancient women's steady and consistent gathering was more conducive to eating on the go. Perhaps this explains why women snack more frequently than men.

Crescendo fasting (two to three days per week) still has benefits of for women – but why? Perhaps, although the gathering by women provided more consistent feeding, there were inevitable periods of caloric scarcity (seasonal variation) which requires females to be capable of *some* stress resistance. On the note of seasonal variation it would be interesting to see (as I found no studies) on whether fasting works more in sync with the female body during colder months. I suspect that there must be some correlation if my suspicion is correct. Men's work was more "dramatic" but also less reliable in a society which lacked the means for preserving food. Gathering was more reliable and consistent than hunting.

OUR PALEO ANCESTORS

Let's refer back to the example of humans in Palaeolithic times. It makes sense that a scarcity of food would provoke the secretion of cortisol as that in itself is in response to stressful situation (potential death) thus motivating people to seek out food.

Common belief has it that hunter-gatherers spent most of their day gathering food for a big meal at night. In his book

Ingalik Social Culture, Cornelius Osgood notes that the Ingalik hunter-gatherers of the interior of Alaska ate only once per day: "As has been made clear, the principal meal and sometimes the only one of the day is eaten in the evening." The Aché hunter-gatherers of Paraguay, according to French anthropologist Pierre Clastres, also hunted during the day and feasted in the evening. Furthermore, according to Canadian anthropologist Richard Borshay Lee, the !Kung of Botswana divided themselves into small groups during the day to explore, hunt and gather through the surrounding ranges and then come back together in the evening to "pool the collected resources for the evening meal".

There has long been discussion about hunter-gatherers and their regular fasting periods. However, recently there has been speculation about the validity of these claims. All the later findings were made in between 1958 and 1972, so perhaps they are slightly outdated. New research, particularly by Anore Jones who wrote a book called *Plants That We Eat*, suggests a completely opposing view about the Iñupiat of north-west Alaska. According to Ms Jones, there is no reason to believe that in normal, warm climates these hunter-gatherers would go through frequent fasting periods. Ms Jones outlines in detail how the Iñupiat people prepare themselves for the winter months. They gather berries and ferment them in seal skin. They also cut marks into the roots of vegetables in the summer time so that they can find them during the colder months.

According to a 2014 study from *Biology Letters*, hunter-gatherers have less famine than agriculturalists. The hypothesis proposes that these hunter-gatherer ancestors adapted to frequent famines, and the "thrifty genotypes" are responsible for today's obesity epidemic. The study used a cross-cultural sample of 186 different cultures. The findings concluded that contrary to common belief it was the agricultural societies which actually went through more frequent periods of fasting and famine. It was only the cold-climate hunter-gatherers who experienced prolonged periods of fasting, but even then we can see that many, such as the previously mentioned Iñupiat, had means to work around this.

I do think that because instances of famine did exist, fasting schedules such as 5:2 (two days per week) may be the closest to our ancestral nature. The 5:2 diet is eating about 500 calories per day for two days of the week. For example you'd eat 2000 per day (if this was what you required) and 500 on Wednesday and Friday. But of course this depends where your ancestors were located in the world. The difference in climate may also pose some interesting questions around the relationship between your ethnic genetic heritage, the proceeding epigenetic inheritance and further predisposition to respond better to more frequent or prolonged fasting schedules. Unfortunately I have not come across any significant research on this topic. The complexity of these historical results means that intermittent fasting is very effective for some and undesirable and ineffective for many others.

THE MAGIC OF REAL FOOD

If someone were to ask you, "What are the nutritional benefits of food?" your answer may be "vitamins and minerals". The classic example is beta-carotene in carrots which is known to help your improve eyesight in the dark; an orange is commonly acknowledged as a great way to boost your immune system. Clearly micronutrients are incredibly important to our health. However, the answer usually lacks one word: fibre.

Many people don't know about the benefits of fibre. Dr Jason Fung describes the role of fibre as a substance which "subtracts rather than adds". If we examine the properties and effects of sugar and insulin levels, fibre is good, despite "subtraction" possibly being interpreted as losing something. Fibre will reduce the absorption of carbohydrates and this has the effect of reducing blood glucose levels and insulin. A study in 2000 from the *New England Journal of Medicine* shows us that patients with type 2 diabetes were fed liquid meals with

55 per cent carbohydrates, some with fibre and some without any dietary fibre added. The results showed that fibre reduces the peak of insulin and blood glucose levels, even though the amount of carbohydrates and calorie levels were the same.

It's clear that increased cortisol and insulin contribute to the obesity risk, and fibre reduces blood glucose and insulin. Therefore we can say that adequate fibre intake is a vital component to a well-balanced diet by reducing an unnatural ratio of these hormones. You could say that fibre subtracts some of the negatives of a high carbohydrate meal. However, this doesn't mean you should rely on fibre supplements and eat potato chips.

What is fascinating is that natural foods, such as oranges, kiwis or apples, have a balance of fibre that evolved over time to ripen at the *perfect* ratio for these hormonal regulations. This is a beautiful phenomenon when you think about it. Nature is made perfect to work in sync with our bodies – and yet we reject it. The toxicity of food doesn't necessarily lie in the food's properties, but rather than in the processing, which can skew the balance and prevent the body receiving the full complement of nutrients.

Our bodies contain satiety hormones (Peptide YY and cholecystokinin) which naturally respond to the consumption of fat and protein. The reason carbohydrates tend to be over-consumed isn't completely because of the carbohydrates, but also the way they are eaten. Imagine trying to eat six oranges. It would be difficult, even though each one only has an average of sixty-two calories. The pulp in the fruit contains fibre (satiety and expanding), creating a feeling of being full. If we compare this to drinking orange juice, the digestion process quickens and therefore blood glucose levels increase. Following this increase, insulin spikes and with this drink comes ease in consuming it. Therefore it becomes easier to overeat this way, even if the orange juice appears to be "healthy". A 2012 research survey from *The Southern Medical Journal* found that one-third of participants who responded believed that juice was at least as healthy as fresh fruit.

When you're not getting enough fibre in your diet, proteins, lipids and sugars are absorbed into the upper intestine. What this means is that bacteria in the gut begin to starve. In order to not starve, these bacteria catabolise the lining of the gut and cause a breakdown of the tissue.

There are two different types of fibre, soluble and insoluble. Both are incredibly important for our health, digestion as well as preventing disease. The best way to ensure you're getting enough fibre is to eat a wide variety of wholefoods. A sign you're doing so is to see whether your plate has a wide variety of colours. Colour in vegetables generally signifies certain concentrations of specific vitamins. For example, dark green vegetables are particularly high in magnesium.

Prebiotics are basically a special form of fibre, found in a wide variety of fruits and vegetables. They are particularly abundant in the skin of plant foods. So think twice before peeling away the skin on your sweet potato or apple. Prebiotics have also been shown to increase brain-derived neurotrophic factor (BDNF) which is a protein which also increases through consumption of antidepressants. Additionally, prebiotics have been shown to reduce cortisol and help with emotional processing.

If you're consuming refined carbohydrates instead of your required fibre intake, you're asking for trouble. Many think that fibre is one thing, when in fact there are different types. There's fibre in plants, in pectin, mushrooms, fruits, onions, garlic – this list goes on. They all feed off different types of bacteria, which is why it's so important to eat a wide variety of sources of fibre. Too much fibre can also be bad, so don't overdo it. Eat 1/4 cup of broccoli, 1/4 cup of carrots 1/4 cup of tomato and 1/4 cup of kale – instead of 1 cup of broccoli.

We know conclusively that sugar is directly linked to cancer. Some studies have shown that refinedsugar aggravates the risk for breast cancer by four times. One packet of some sort of "natural fruit candy" usually has over 20 g of sugar, around the RDA for the average adult. It's hidden everywhere. Too much sugar is going to cause your body fat to redistribute from subcutaneous to visceral and liver deposits. You want fat under the skin, not in your liver and around your organs.

Vinegar and Blood Sugar

There are other substances which have a remarkable impact on the levels of blood insulin and glucose. Vinegar consumption has been shown in multiple studies to compensate for the spike of insulin after a meal full of carbohydrates. (I still remember the look on my friend's face as I took shots of apple cider vinegar.)

A 2005 study from the *European Journal of Clinical Nutrition* has shown that supplementation with vinegar lowers the glucose and insulin response and this increases feelings of satiety after a meal high in carbohydrates. It should be noted that this hypothesis is based on products which contain acetic acid. The level of acetic acid in vinegar is the specific variable which had a positive correlation with the satiety rating of participants. Most organic apple cider vinegars contain acetic acid, but be sure to double check if you are purchasing it for this specific reason.

So...if you make the mistake of going to McDonald's, ask for pickles on your cheeseburger.

Reducing Cortisol

Stress will always be part of our lives. Elevated stress levels will also make it extremely difficult to make virtuous decisions, as stress really does make you vulnerable to the temptation of hedonistic behaviour. Distress will often lead to a mindset of seeking compensation through short-term pleasure.

Before we move on, I would like to make a brief disclosure

on my attack on cortisol. Cortisol serves various functions in the body which are beneficial, or else we wouldn't have it in the first place! In chaotic and dangerous situations, cortisol improves our ability to stay active and alert. However, as I've made clear, we live in a world that cultivates an abundance of *unnecessary* stresses to the extent where it's imperative for us to frequently and consistently understand how to manage it. Below are some adaptogenic herbs for cortisol reduction. *Adaptogenic* means they do not alter mood but stabilise physiological process and promote homeostasis. The relevant example is decreasing the body's cellular sensitivity to stress. Many of these herbs have been used both in ancient and modern times. There are plenty more but I selected the following for two reasons: quality of evidence and also my own personal use.

Ten adaptogenic herbs for reducing cortisol:

1. Bacopa *(Bacopa monnieri)*
2. Ginkgo *(ginkgo biloba)*
3. Arctic root *(Rhodiola rosea)*
4. Ashwagandha *(Withania somnifera)*
5. Holy basil *(Ocimum sanctum* or *Ocimum tenuiflorum)*
6. Schisandra *(Schisandra chinensis)*
7. Maca *(Lepidium meyenii)*
8. Eleuthero *(Eleutherococcus senticosus)*
9. Astragalus root *(Astragalus propinquus)*
10. Jiaogulan *(Gynostemma pentaphyllum*)

You can also supplement magnesium, specifically magnesium glycerinate. Supplementing vitamin D3 (especially during the winter months) is useful.

Supplements, adaptogenic herbs and other methods such as massage, wholefoods and anti-inflammatory diets, spending time in nature or even acupuncture – these are just a few of the many things you can try to reduce cortisol in the short term. However, don't take a certain supplement (especially synthetic ones) and rely on them. The best way to reduce cortisol is to get to the cause. The brain can be changed.

NEUROPLASTICITY AND MINDFULNESS

Neuroplasticity, also known as brain plasticity, is a term used to describe change, often intentional, that occurs over the course of an individual's life. Before the latter half of the twentieth century there was an adamant belief that changes made in the brain during childhood dictate a static state of the brain for a lifetime. Neuroplasticity opposes this and shows us that our brains have the capacity to change (hence the term *plastic*), even during adulthood. The brain can change and this change is quantifiable.

In a well-known study from *IEEE Signal Processing Magazine* in 2008, Davidson and colleague Antoine Lutz explored the idea that "meditation is fundamentally no different than other forms of skill acquisition that can induce plastic changes in the brain". Tibetan Buddhist monks (who had meditated for thousands of hours over the course of their lives) were recruited through the help of the Dalai Lama after his speech at the Society for Neuroscience's annual meeting in Washington DC. The research on these participants has shown that through countless hours of meditation the structural composition of their brain has quite literally changed.

Neuroplasticity has given researchers grounds to track how meditation, even within short periods of time, increases grey matter and cortical thickness in several areas of the brain. Increased grey matter was found in the prefrontal cortex. This area is responsible for functions such as problem solving, planning and emotional regulation. With increased thickness of the cortex comes the improved ability to control learning, memory, depression and – most importantly for this discussion – stress.

The answer is clear – we need to decrease our stress levels, not only for our body composition but for our peace of mind.

As listed previously, there are various herbs and supplements that perhaps work at reducing cortisol. Sitting in front of the television may be mistaken as stress relief, but I see it as stagnation and procrastination (and as I mentioned before, after age twenty-five your life shortens 21.8 minutes for every hour slouched in front of the television). Entertainment is an escape and does not actively achieve anything other than avoidance of the issue. If your stress levels are high, it's vital to take *active* measures to reduce them. It's critical for everybody to understand how to manage their own stress, without the use of pharmaceutical drugs. Stress can quickly debilitate and create strong dependency.

There is a solution to stress that does not require you to take anything external, or to numb your mind with distractions. This solution places no burden on you financially and, most importantly, is everlasting and cumulative. I'm talking about *mindfulness*.

Many of us watch television, watch videos or even play computer games while we eat. This is called *distracted eating*. It's a bad idea. We surround ourselves with so much stimulation. Eating should be done by itself, because the act itself involves every single sense. When you eat, just eat. When you read, just read. Train yourself to be mindful and attentive to the task you're doing. Make sure to eat *slowly*. Eating slowly is important for:

- Learning temperance and self-control.
- To allow the brief moments for your stomach to signal to your brain that you are full.
- Chewing a lot before you swallow is also important as it will reduce the amount of oxygen the brain requires to digest the food, allowing for greater cognitive acuity.

A 2013 meta-analysis of twenty-four studies from the *American Journal of Clinical Nutrition* looked at the effect of food intake on memory and also the awareness of eating. The studies came together to point towards attentive eating influencing food intake. The act of attentive eating, being mindful and eating slowly is a novel approach for weight loss, exclusive of counting calories. Furthermore, it's important to understand that you must be aware – or mindful – of the reason you are hungry in the first place. Are you physiologically hungry? Or are you hungry in order to compensate for being anxious, or stressed, or worried?

Practise mindfulness through meditative practices to understand the "space between stimulus and response", to quote author, psychiatrist and Holocaust survivor Victor Frankl. This is why fasting is so powerful psychologically – it forces you to confront what is creating hunger, rather than giving you the opportunity to compensate for something by stimulating yourself with food.

The most convincing source I have come across in my research on mindfulness as a means to decrease stress-provoked eating was a 2011 study from the *Journal of Obesity*. This study was based on the knowledge that distress and increased cortisol secretion is directly related to increased fat in the abdominal area. The subjects were overweight and obese women. Over a four-month intervention, researchers kept a close eye on how mindfulness affected the women's behaviours, as well their cortisol awakening response (CAR). Their abdominal fat was monitored using a dual-energy X-ray absorptiometry before the four-month period and after. CAR is the natural secretion of the stress hormone upon waking. The women showed very significant reductions in the hormone after waking and, from this, a decrease in abdominal fat. This study is important as it shows us very clearly the strength of the connection which most have always anecdotally attributed to stress and fat loss. Less cortisol is going to accompany less insulin and less binging/emotional eating due to stress and theoretically a lower risk of obesity.

Just as *eudaimonia* cannot be created through swallowing a pill, neither can control over stress. There are only two options for this: change the environment that is creating the stress; or learn how to manage your stress.

> "Man is not worried by real problems so much as by his imagined anxieties about real problems."
>
> – Epictetus

We've all felt the beauty of the universe – we've heard the waves, the birds chirping, the wind blowing. We've all experienced those moments of peace and wholeness with our surroundings, which the Stoics called *sympatheia*. The French philosopher Pierre Hadot referred to this as *oceanic feeling*. It is the experience of belonging to something larger. It's a realisation that we are an infinitesimal single point in the immensity of the universe – something I call "cosmic goosebumps" or "present energy".

To understand what "present energy" is, or to experience *sympatheia*, you must stop *trying* to "be present". Ironically, when you try to focus, you can't – it's impossible. The *attempt* is proof you have already lost.

The notion of *sympatheia* is a common theme in Stoicism. Chrysippus believed that various parts of the universe held a close affinity with one another. Posidonius, according to many scholars, fully developed this during the end of the second and beginning of the first century BC. The cosmos, in which we experience *sympatheia*, is held together through *tonos (tension)* which is created by *pneuma* ("breath" or "spirit") through fire and air. Pneuma sustains everything. It is our own soul when we pay attention and we are attentive to the present energy of the world. Unfortunately, we escape this state too often. This universal unconsciousness we all share, this anxious haze which consumes so many people in the bustling movement of urbanism leaves a constant stress and ache on the body and the mind.

TEA FOR THE MIND; TEA FOR THE BODY

> "Drink your tea slowly and reverently, as if it is the axis on which the world earth revolves – slowly, evenly, without rushing toward the future. Live the actual moment. Only this moment is life."
>
> – Thich Nhat Hanh

I drink tea for the soothing effect. After reading *The Art of Power,* by Vietnamese Buddhist monk and author Thich Nhat Hanh, I gained an appreciation and a greater understanding of why tea is a symbol of serenity for so many cultures and religions. I understand why tea is so often poeticised, and why it holds a deeper meaning than simply the liquid itself. There's something special in the specific act of drinking (and making) tea and we can use it as practice of mindfulness (which the Stoics call *prosochē*).

When drinking tea we give ourselves the opportunity to activate every sensory experience of our body. Of course, too much tea can be a bad thing; I'm not pressuring you into becoming a tea addict. But, as modern Stoic author Erik Wiegardt said, "Both tea and alcohol affect the nervous system, but on opposite ends of a polarity." And as the Manchuria proverb goes: "You won't see a good drunk in a teahouse."

The numerous health benefits of tea, especially green tea, have been documented for years. Like fruit and vegetables, tea contains polyphenols, mostly in the form of flavonoids. Polyphenols are known to lower the risk of heart disease and are an important medicinal treatment in traditional Chinese medicine. However, *tea* is a very general term and so many tea connoisseurs will only consider black, white, green, oolong and pu-erh as legitimate. All these types come from the *Camellia sinensis* plant, a shrub originating from China and India.

Loose-leaf tea brewed and left for five minutes produces a greater benefit from its antioxidant properties. I like to spend five minutes doing something like stretching or push-ups while my tea brews. Tea isn't restricted just to drinking. To give just one example, you can use tea bags on your eyes to reduce fatigue, which is useful when staring at a screen for a long time (I highly recommend you try this).

The most potent antioxidant in tea is the catechin epigallocatechin gallate (ECGC), which is often marketed as a herbal supplement. ECGC may help fight against free radicals that can contribute to cancer, heart disease and clogged arteries. Some data is encouraging that some teas, specifically green tea, have cancer preventive effects. Black tea may also have similar effects. Evidence from studies into metabolic and cardiovascular health is quite convincing in the benefits about regular tea consumption.

Something I found interesting in my research was that tea has actually been associated with a lower risk of depression. Whether this is because of the mindful and attentive nature of drinking it, or the caffeine, or the amino acid *L-Theanine*, is unknown. A meta-analysis in 2005 of eleven studies showed that overall nearly 23,000 participants found for every three servings of tea consumed per day the rate of depression fell by 37 per cent.

Beware that there are over 400 chemicals in tea, some of which can have adverse reactions with certain drugs. Although the effects of tea could be said to be surprising, remember that they don't cure disease. But there's no harm in consuming tea as it is simply a form of increasing fluid intake, connects you to your surroundings and acts as a "responsible" choice when you've had one too many cups of coffee. Despite popular belief, tea – or even coffee for that matter – won't dehydrate you when drunk in moderation. Caffeine only becomes a problem when you increase it over around 5-6 mg per kilogram. Anything below this and most studies show that the water you consume with the beverage compensates for any loss. Ireland, Iran and most noteworthy of all, Turkey (where people drink on average 16.6 pounds of tea annually) have life expectancies that make clear the connection between longevity and tea consumption. Of course this doesn't include socio-economic status or how the tea is being consumed. (This flaw is well portrayed by the English proverb: "A man without a moustache is like a cup of tea without sugar.")

Don't expect to live to 100 by over-consuming tea! But this soothing drink is something I will always associate with health. My grandmother, who is nearly 100 now (touch wood), drinks copious amounts of tea (known as *chai* in Iran). Anecdotal? Sure – so take this with a grain of salt (but not in your tea – yuck!).

ANALYTICAL MEDITATIONS

Are you uncomfortable with the idea that your thoughts aren't your own? Your thoughts are merely a reflection of the exterior, but we experience them on the interior. This may feel invasive, penetrating, almost frightening; such an epiphany is poisonous to the ego. But it is this bittersweet epiphany we must embrace in order to be truly free, fulfilled and connect with our inner *eudaimonia*.

One of my favourite analogies is what I call "learning to swim". The water flowing in a stream represents your constant flow of thoughts, ideas, insights and conceptualisations which are, whether you believe it or not, out of your control. No matter what you do, unless the stream is blocked (equating to death), the water will continue to flow. Most people live their lives inside the river and so they get wet; they don't know how to swim and so they are defined by their thoughts. Stoics,

Buddhists, Taoists and Stoics step on to the side of the stream as a non-judgemental spectator and they had to learn how to swim in order to get there. As Seneca said, "We are more often frightened than hurt; and we suffer more from imagination than from reality."

Buddhist teaching revolves around ending suffering and stepping outside the cycle of reincarnation. Although Buddhism and Stoicism differ in some aspects, there are parallels, and so they are worthy of comparison. For Stoics, reasoning is emphasised for one's identity and expression of moral excellence. For Buddhists it is breaking the cycle of reincarnation. The cycle is broken as one becomes enlightened – enlightenment being a state in which an individual understands the truth about life (perhaps equivalent to sagehood, the Stoic moral ideal.)

Buddhism is much more perceptual and requires periods of intentional solitude and retreat. Meditation isn't practised to actually gain anything; rather it is practised to lose what one doesn't need – anger, anxiety, frustration, stress, depression and the fear of death. To the Buddhist, these are factors of the mind which must be lost in order to fulfil the purpose of their journey. This is to be overcome through consistent practice of meditation.

In Zen Buddhism, *zazen* meditation literally translates to "seated meditation". Within this style of meditation there are three aspects, according to Philip Kapleau's book, *Three Pillars of Zen*. The aim of the first (*shikantaza* meditation) is to focus on the sound and motions of your breath. Tthe aim of the second (concentration meditation) is to allow your thoughts to come in as they usually would, but as with the stream analogy, instead of recognising them as your own, learn to recognise them as existing, but not defining you.

There is also a third, rather fascinating, type of meditation called *koan* introspections. *Koan*s are cryptic paradoxical questions which supersede logical and rational plains of thought. The introspection is then to resolve this irrational paradox. Master Hakuin Ekaku (1686-1768), who was one of the most influential figures in Japanese Zen Buddhism, is often cited for his famous *koan* given to students: "You know the sound of two hands clapping; tell me, what is the sound of one hand clapping?" There is no answer; there is no epiphany relating to an objective answer. After months of contemplating the irrationality the student comes to an enlightened recognition of the absurdity of the *koan* and then "shifts up" in the journey. Perhaps *koan* introspections are similar to negative visualisations – both are based on linguistic frameworks, although clearly *koan*s are far from being rational and analytical.

Negative visualisation is a Stoic meditation in which you intentionally conjure pessimistic thought in order to improve appreciation and gratefulness. The way I like to see it is being mindful of your own pessimism, so you can figure out what the hell to actually do with it when it isn't voluntary.

Many Buddhist meditations help a person become more mindful. In Stoicism, *prosochē* – a term coined by Epictetus – is the term for mindfulness. *Prosochē* is vigilance and critical self-awareness to the self on the path to wisdom. Donald Robertson describes this concept as "continual self-monitoring of one's thoughts and actions, as they happen, in the here and now". Despite the differences between Stoicism and Buddhism, the parallels centre around this idea of attention to your surroundings. Stoic author Elen Buzaré tells us that Stoic mindfulness is similar to two Buddhist meditations, *Samatha* and *Vipassana*. *Samatha* is practised by calming the mind (*citta*) and mental impressions (*sankhāra*). *Vipassana* (insight) is about understanding the true nature of reality through three marks of existence: impermanence, suffering and actualisation. Pāli canon explains that the Buddha never tells us *Vipassana* and *Samatha* are mutually exclusive. They are two "qualities of the mind" conjured through meditation. One calms the mind to lead to insight, and vice versa. They interact and are inclusive of each other.

To a Stoic it doesn't make sense to not think about anything. Stoic mindfulness is explicitly analytical. Pierre Hadot suggests that Stoic mindfulness includes "the memorisation and assimilation of the fundamental dogmas and rules of life". Some psychologists may call Stoic mindfulness "flow"; I see it as simply being congruent in the sense that your thoughts and everything about you aligns together with your current actions. To practise attention or mindfulness, you can simply ask yourself, "What are you doing?" I suggest integrating your *prosoche* first and foremost simply while we are waiting for sleep, as Seneca recommends. As long as we're alive, the minutes before sleep will always be there.

In addition, pinpoint regular activities in your life where you find yourself especially drawn to being vigilant and self-aware of your moral character. An example could be drinking tea, which we spoke about before, tending to the garden, writing, playing basketball, yoga, etc. Take your time, breathe and relax into the activity you're doing so that you lose track of time, thoughts of past or future. Simply be in frequency, essentially tune your brain to the frequency of the radio station (the activity you're doing) so you have a strong signal and you don't miss one moment.

The key I've found is to relax into *that* which came before your birth, exists during your life and will always exist after your death, when you pull your motives and actions through this source. Here you will find tranquillity, and here you will bring out your most rational self.

Question your very actions at this moment, not as a means to arouse internal antagonism and distress but in order to rationalise *what* you are doing. We all have an internal narrator within us; make his job easy and have him simply explain your actions to you in a pragmatic and non-judgemental way. Remember that there are just facts and nothing else. Practise and reaffirm this repeatedly, to solidify attention as your founding state of mind. Resistance will be inevitable for those unaccustomed to practising this.

Through years of trial, error, study and becoming more conscious, I began to understand that most of what we perceive to be pain is actually thoughts that stay with us and latch on. It's not necessarily the substance and quality of the thoughts themselves. But over time these thoughts can become warped and deluded, and this is what buries them deep into the soul. Sometimes you may lack the ability to perceive your thoughts for their rational significance. It is not the experience that is damaging and fatiguing to our mind and body, it is our frustration with the fact that these thoughts follow us like a shadow. Thoughts can be so convincing. When we are wet in the stream, we feel the wetness, but we forget that it is possible for us to learn to swim at any moment, at any age, whenever we make the decision to.

I am not against meditation in the sense that you set aside a period each day to focus on your breathing. I've done this before plenty of times and it's awesome, but this should not be your primary goal, in my humble opinion. I see potential in solitude for growth, but I also see potential for comfort being formed in a habit which may reinforce the idea that mindfulness and presence is exclusive to solitude. Now, this will vary for different people, so please do not take this perspective as an absolute; but for the Stoic, it simply serves no good to isolate oneself in this manner. If you are going to do the tradi-tional type of meditation – seated, with your legs crossed – a great idea is to take this practice outside to a public park, somewhere where you're not confining yourself. Mindfulness, as with *Vipassana*, is "getting to the point" as you practice it throughout everyday actives, in the eye of the storm.

Mindfulness meditation increases grey matter in the right frontal cortex. Increased activity in the left prefrontal cortex is associated with changes in happiness and mood. Different meditative practices can produce different effects on the brain, although many overlap. Regardless, what's fascinating is that simply doing these practices each day literally changes the structure of the brain.

Epictetus warns us of the danger of losing the momentum of *prosochē*. He says, "Because of your fault today your affairs must be necessarily in a worse condition on future occasions." It is our consistent *prosochē* to present actions, desires and impressions which, at the end of our life, define how happy we are. True *prosochē* takes vigilance, self-awareness and rigidity of the mind. Focus your *prosochē* on the journey itself rather than the end goal. Epictetus tells us: "So, is it possible to be altogether faultless? No, that is impracticable." To be happy is to be happy with the progression, without any real expectation of the result.

LACKING COMMAND

> "If you accomplish something good with hard work, the labour passes quickly, but the good endures; if you do something shameful in pursuit of pleasure, the pleasure passes quickly, but the shame endures."
>
> – Musonius Rufus

AKRASIA

Hyperbolic discounting refers to the tendency for people to choose a smaller and more immediate reward over a larger but prolonged reward. Over time, as we ignore long-term rewards, they lose their ability to make us act. We lose our ability to self-govern the rational approach and therefore we more frequently fall victim to a paradigm of short-term gratification. Financially, this might mean using credit cards instead of saving in incremental amounts. With health, this might mean choosing soda over water, or browsing Reddit instead of working out.

The idea of hyperbolic discounting goes back to the era of Socrates and Plato. The Greek word *akrasia* means "lacking command" or "lacking self-control", and describes anything against reasonable judgement.

Socrates, in Plato's *Protogoras*, questions how being *akratic* is even possible. Socrates was perplexed at why an individual would ever choose option B if option A is clearly the most rational and objective choice. Furthermore, in the dialogue of *Protogoras*, Socrates proclaims that *akrasia* in fact does not exist because "no one goes willingly toward the bad". He is saying that in any given situation, if an individual decides to act in a specific way (which may be perceived as being "bad), it was determined to be good as "to him it seemed so". This action is actively pursued, as good is man's natural goal. Euripides, a tragedian of Athens, said, "I am overcome by evil, and I realise what evil I am about to do, but my passion controls my plans."

If our soul is rational by nature, then, as Socrates said, how could it do otherwise than what it judges to be best?

Too much opinion in the moment and not enough thinking will put you in a bad situation. You need to constantly be asking yourself questions to raise your self-awareness.

Prosochē: *"What are you doing?"*

Firstly, we can approach hyperbolic discounting by practising mindfulness and being attuned to the present moment. When we have *prosochē* and we ask ourselves, "What am I doing?" we quickly become aware of our surroundings. To quote Victor Frankl: "Between stimulus and response there is a space. In that space is our power to choose our response. In our response lies our growth and our freedom." We spend most of our lives in an unconscious state, simply acting and being immersed in the experience. When we ask ourselves, "What am I doing?" we place ourselves in an advantageous position. Yet it is often not enough to be aware and attentive to this space between stimulus and response, because what's stopping you from closing the space?

Contemplation: *"Why are you doing this?"*

By thinking, contemplating and questioning the intent and consequence of your actions in combination with *prosochē*, you are able to understand the relationship between your short-term (what are you doing?) and long-term (why are you doing this?) selves. Through enforcing a need to think critically about your actions, even though they may seem insignificant, you give yourself the benefit of reinforcing awareness between both modes. I understand this may seem a bit "woo-woo" and mystical, but bear with me. We can compare this to an argument. If you wish to argue well and with reason, you must understand both sides of the argument. If you understand the reason for someone else's position more than your own, but you still hold firm to your own argument, then surely this is correct if you are basing your judgements on reason. If you understand when both of these personas of the mind are conflicting, then you can better allow for interchange between them both in favour of reason and action.

THINKING IN THIRD PERSON

You must develop a vision for what your life would be like if you were living optimally, in good health and with peace of mind. This vision should not be something as nonsensical as "a six-pack", as this is not sophisticated enough to be self-sustaining. In forming this vision, treat yourself as if you are observing someone you don't know but wish to help. Prescribe the best course of action to cultivate this vision with the tools and resources available. Now, this may seem easy but perhaps you are ambivalent about whether this person should be around in the first place. As someone who used to play a lot of computer games, I like to see this character as one in a game who I am attempting to level up. I ask you to take a third-person glance because often we are capable of under-standing what another person needs to do for themselves; but when it comes to ourselves, we may have a blind spot. Now break down this person you are observing into three possible directions:

1. The **best** possible outcome.

2. The **worst** possible outcome.

3. The **current** direction.

With the decisions and habits you have right now, in which direction is this person heading? There are only two directions; a man is either living a life just or unjust.

How do you determine your current direction?

Write down everything you do for one typical, average day.

For each activity, multiply it by 365 days.

For each activity, ask yourself: What will be the result of doing this 365 days a year?

If **just**, *how* can you improve?

If **unjust**, *where* do you go from here?

Let's take the example of an individual who, after living a good life, has experienced the death of a loved one. He then falls back into his previous vice-driven pursuits. Pleasure becomes the solution for the sigh of "what's the point anyway?" This aligns well with the phrase "once a smoker, always a smoker". A previous "lane" which was once explored has been redis-covered due to lack of clear direction. And so the individual's suffering begins again.

MAN'S SEARCH FOR MEANING

A belief in the meaninglessness of life and pleasure-seeking go hand in hand to sustain someone. It's as if we naturally require discomfort to live life, and for some this discomfort is based on substances and habits. Meaning in life comes from having a purpose you attach yourself to. This could be anything. Sometimes it's a worthy purpose and other times it's one which leads you in the wrong direction. Regardless, having one gives you drive and ambition.

Logotherapy was developed by Viktor Frankl. Logotherapy is a frame of psychology which was popularised through Dr Frankl's book *Man's Search for Meaning*, written in 1946. This inspiring book chronicles his experience in concentration camps during World War II. Dr Frankl cultivated logotherapy in order to feel content despite the outcome, immersing in the positivity of his purpose and maintaining his presence and peace of mind in moments where most people would fall apart. It's a great advantage to have a *logo*, a purpose to live for, which you can fall back on in times where impressions and temptations get in the way of making the rational, and more long-term, decision. Just as an example, your *logo* could be to be a great father and raise kind children. Even if you're not a father yet, your goal may be to develop your character now in your youth to emulate the figure you would want these kind children to look up to in their adolescence. This purpose can be a saviour to the pause between stimuli and response where you question your actions. Life really is defined in these brief moments and so we should take them much more seriously than their length in seconds.

Picture a map on a new video game you buy. When new, none of the map has been discovered yet. As you uncover new areas of the map they become visible on the saved map that we refer back to for direction. These maps are never forgotten on the console's memory card. It is the same for our memories. Subconsciously we have always mapped out these "lanes" as we have travelled there before. The fewer lanes we have travelled the fewer we have, and thus the more familiar and comforting it can be to go our own biases. But it's exciting to go to untouched areas on the map. You have to discover more of the map in order to free yourself of the comfort in going in only one or two directions. It's the only way you can "clock the game".

If we look at the successful wise man, he has lived through times of vice and discovered all the wrong areas of the map, but now he knows where these areas of vice are and he can instead move in the right direction.

Understand where each trajectory is going to take you and re-affirm to yourself that a direction will either take you up or down, to heaven or hell, to good or bad, towards light or darkness and do this with every action you take. If this attentiveness to the present moment is practised enough, in conjunction with asking yourself "why am I doing this?" you will solidify your boundaries. The "hey, no, you shouldn't be doing that" voice in your head tells you what matters. This is the little spark of rationality we are all born with. The truth is undesirable and honesty is too often punished. In today's world this rationale is like a rock which needs repeated mining to bring out the ore which is of value. Anxiety, fear, distrust of your own temperance and anything "bad" can help you do good. Negative experiences are only your enemies if they are working against you, but they are powerful if you have them positioned correctly.

PART SIX:
DAWN TO DUSK

"At dawn, when you have trouble getting out of bed, tell yourself, 'I have to go to work - as a human being. What do I have to complain of, if I'm going to do what I was born for – the things I was brought into the world to do? Or is this what I was created for? To huddle under the blankets and stay warm?'"

– Marcus Aurelius

MORNING PREMEDITATIONS

Remaining in the comfort of your bed's warmth in the hours of sunrise is tempting to say the least. The feeling of the comfortable cocoon of bed sheets and the world at your fingertips through your phone may be a pleasant experience. Frequently this becomes a debilitating tone set for the rest of the day.

How do you face the day when this temptation is too strong? What do you do if you want to get up, but your mind isn't prepared and accepting of the outer world? To premeditate is to prepare our minds and bodies for the life of the day with vigour and no contempt for the outside world, but to embrace it with conviction, enforcing upon ourselves our expectation of the worst possibilities. Through premeditations we prepare our minds for the potential negative events that may come by leaving the comfort of the bed. If this is done right, the urge to stay in bed will cease to exist from the very moment your thoughts enter this realm of contemplation.

Marcus Aurelius reminds us, "Begin each day by telling yourself: today I will be meeting with interference, ingratitude, insolence, disloyalty, ill will, and selfishness – all of them due to the offenders' ignorance of what is good and what is evil." Recognise that interference, ingratitude, insolence and every other emotional or physical burden is part of reality, not something that can be avoided through burying yourself under your quilt. The moment you wake up, flood your conscious thoughts with the expectation that today may be your very last day. Vocalise this. If you remain in your introspective safe space, how do you expect to overcome adversity and discomfort as the day progresses? Ask yourself, "Can your comfort realistically be enjoyed by first finding comfort in the pleasure of warmth?" Just as you should make your bed in the morning, so you should make your mind.

We look at another person's suffering as a means to rationalise our own and remain unattached. We must also apply this approach as we wake up from sleep and enter back into our sober senses. Nightmares and bad dreams are simply that, nightmares and bad dreams that bothered you while you were asleep. In your waking hours, perceive events and situations just as you would these dreams, which don't exist anymore. Find an image you can hang, an art work, a song or any object which aligns itself with the quotation above from Marcus Aurelius or a similar message. Find something that reminds you of the shortness of life. Take time to find this and make sure that it truly gives justice to this message. Find a way to become aware of this message in your waking moments immediate, as

a reminder. Keep a journal and write down your thoughts –
this is essential to preserve a mindset of rigidity.

Something I like to sketch and ponder on is Hierocles'
circle. You begin by thinking [or in this case drawing] about
yourself, your family, your friends, your neighbourhood, your
city, country, humanity, the universe itself. I meditate on this in
times when I am resisting the unpleasant or things feel out of
control. For some reason this meditation helps me recalibrate
my equanimity and focus and gives me perspective.

Think back to yesterday. What do you actually remember?
As human beings we only truly remember vivid details in the
events which are out of the ordinary. If something frightening
or startling occurs, we remember this; if something saddens us,
we remember it. Striking events are preserved in our memory
with clarity. So many of the small and seemingly insignificant
moments we experience throughout every waking second of
the day are ignored and these are what compound over time to
long-lasting and significant change, as Zeno reminds us.

When you write things down, you can preserve the small
details and examine what actually compounds to larger change
over time. You will be giving yourself the ability to see your
actions, what works for you, what doesn't work and what
actually comes prior to unfavourable consequences. By writing
you appreciate the small things that matter, but which your
mind forgets. Get into the habit of writing early in the morning
– this will give you a greater sense of peace moving forward
into the day. Trust me on this. Write down what you're grateful
for and how you'll be better today. It's such an important habit
that is overlooked.

"Begin at once to live, and count each separate
day as a separate life."

– Seneca.

We get busy, we live frantic and chaotic lives, but if we remain honest about our thoughts, actions and deepest selves we are then able to maintain our focus on virtue as we move through the day. Marcus Aurelius warns us: "[Don't] let your imagination be crushed by life as a whole. Don't try to picture everything bad that could possibly happen. Stick with the situation at hand." Always have somebody in your life whose way of life mirrors the character which you wish to embody. In every situation where you doubt your ability to live in virtue, mirror their mind, actions and words. It's critical to always have someone you admire and this way you will make the correct decisions more often.

Ask yourself: "What would they do if they didn't want to get out of bed"? Would the person I am striving to emulate feel bad for himself and not take advantage of another day being alive?".

Of course not!

Here's a Russian proverb I'll leave you with to finish this section.

"Morning wiser than evening".

THE SCIENCE OF SLEEP

Without sleep, we end up sleep-deprived. We've all been there; perhaps you're sleep-deprived right now. Being sleep-deprived places a huge toll on your psychological well-being. It's also a stressor that directly stimulates the release of cortisol and activities the body's sympathetic nervous system. In 1910, adults slept an average of nine hours per day – much higher than many people today would ever dream (no pun intended) of reaching on a consistent basis. For the average human being, 37–45 per cent higher cortisol levels are often reported in the evening after being sleep-deprived.

In 2016, the Centers for Disease Control and Prevention analysed 2014 data from the Behavioral Risk Factor Surveillance

System. The survey questioned 444,306 people in the United States on their normal sleeping habits. The results concluded that 11.8 per cent reported less than five hours, while only 4.4 per cent reported nine hours of sleep, which used to be the *average* in 1910. Furthermore only 65.2 per cent reported getting the amount of sleep that is recommended as healthy (this number is 64.9 per cent if we take into account the age-adjusted prevalence). In the past our average time spent asleep was longer than it is today and over the last century it has been quickly declining as we adopt a new way of life.

Leptin and ghrelin are two key hormones responsible for regulation of appetite, based on your specific schedule of eating. This regular pattern is impacted when sleep becomes sporadic. Decreased leptin and increased ghrelin are both directly associated with weight gain. Increased cortisol and ghrelin, along with decreased leptin and sleep deprivation, leads to increased consumption of food. The more fat cells you have the more oestrogen you produce – oestrogen being the female sex hormone (which men have too in smaller amounts).

There have been noticeable trends in girls getting their periods earlier, around age nine or ten. Paediatric and adolescent gynaecologist Dr Julie Powell sees three reasons for this occurring: obesity, chemical exposure, and social and psychological stress. I guess the early hours school children are made to wake up in addition to the xenoestrogens (artificial hormones which mimic the function of oestrogen) found in additives of food, plus the increase in body fat globally and other social and psychological stresses, all come together in an exacerbating manner, giving girls their periods at younger ages.

Although boys are reaching puberty at earlier rates than before (not to the drastic extent girls are), it's clear obese boys develop slightly later than others. The reasoning then goes that the increased levels of oestrogen in their body is one of the main causes of this phenomenon.

So leptin is very important for weight loss and it's now

widely accepted that those who have difficulty losing weight have a leptin resistance, meaning the signalling for your appetite is not working correctly. You've probably noticed your appetite is different when you're not sleeping correctly (while travelling, for example). When the brain cannot receive the leptin signal then the body is presumed to be starving and thus the desire to eat increases, and we become stagnant and sedentary as a survival adaptation to conserve energy. This leads to the couch potato scenario which your "evolutionary self" is applauding.

WHY DO WE SLEEP?

Approximately one-third of our life is spent asleep. There is no single reason for why we sleep – at least, researchers haven't yet found it.. Sleep is an experience where things get a bit mysterious. We can study sleep, we can observe it, we can even understand it through neuroscience. But sleep is part of the human experience that nobody has been able to completely understand.

Think about it: for hours each night we blast off into another realm where our subconscious takes us on a ride where we undoubtedly experience a loss of ego and sense of self. My favourite example is of a friend of mine, Alex, who speaks about flying through mountains during his sleep; an absurd concept when you really think about it, but it's something so many people experience every night.

What is it about sleep that creates such odd experiences so foreign to our everyday nature? Why is it that our subconscious defies what is physically possible when we're asleep? It's these sorts of human experiences that many philosophical, spiritual and religious ideas are born from, in my humble opinion. It's in these moments where we are able to experience a glimpse of something arguably not constructed by us. Perhaps this humbling experience allows us to become open to the possibility that something exists beyond our comprehension. But this experience isn't the defining truth of the nature of sleep;

it is the conclusion that we form from this which is important. For instance, sleep to the Stoic is not aligned with the view of Animists who propose that there is no true distinction between the material and spiritual world. Animists believe the soul is detached from the body during sleep, while a Stoic sees the urge to shut your eyes as a weakening of the spirit, not out of ill health, but out of the simple requirement for physiological and psychological rest.

Over the last century multiple theories have argued about the reasons for sleep. If we look to the animal kingdom we see that most animals sleep, except for very rare exceptions such as dolphins and bullfrogs who simply *rest*. All animals experience a drop in their metabolic rate while sleeping. When asleep the body doesn't require as much energy as it needs for the bustling movement of the day.

One of the earliest theories of sleep is called *adaptive inactivity*, which considers that sleep is a function based on an animal's specific ecological niche. Their sleeping pattern is founded on the need to conserve energy and survive through certain periods of the twenty-four-hour day. For instance, an animal that hunts at night conserves their energy during the day. Humans consolidate energy during the night and hunt during the day with the modern weapon, the credit card. Sleep researcher Ian Oswald suggests that the different types of sleep humans experience correspond to the various restoration processes. Rapid eye movement (REM) sleep is responsible for our brain's growth and repair, while wave sleep is more useful for the restoration of the body. Growth hormone is released, which is important for the repair of muscular tissue. Another sleep researcher, J.A. Horne, extends this theory and suggests that sleep is divided into core or *essential* sleep and also *optimal* sleep.

It's important to note that despite multiple theories being argued for sleep, this doesn't mean they are necessarily mutually exclusive. The adaptive inactivity evolutionary theory aligns itself well with the fact that other theorists argue for synaptic homeostasis. The brain picks and chooses the synaptic connections made during the day to essentially "filter" the needed or the unneeded cognitive synaptic pathways during rest. This allows us to hunt, gather and escape from predators efficiently during wakefulness to secure a greater chance of survival. Both theories are somewhat complementary to each other.

In mammals the "control room" is located in the suprachiasmatic nuclei (SCN) of the hypothalamus region of the brain. This nuclei is highly responsive to the stimuli of light and dark. According to research from *Progress in Molecular Biology and Translational Science* in 2013 and the *Proceedings of the National Academy of Sciences* in 2009 the circadian clock can disrupt overall energy balance and increase the risk of certain chronic diseases when desynchronised from other peripheral circadian clocks (e.g., similar peripheral clocks in liver tissue). Furthermore, it has been hypothesised by a study on time-restricted feeding on mice from *Cell Metabolism* in 2012 that certain fasting regimes can impose a diurnal rhythm for food consumption and this can then improve the gene expression from regular rhythms. This means that fasting regimes allow us the possibility of reprogramming the molecular mechanisms behind body weight regulation and the metabolism.

According to 2014 research from *Sleep Medicine*, eating very late at night reduces the quality of your sleep. A meta-analysis coming out of the *Journal of Sleep Research* in 2009 proposed that very late eaters run the risk of disrupting their normal sleep patterns. Organisms evolved over time to restrict their hunting and gathering activities to either night or day through a circadian clock, so certain processes occur at the optimal moment in time.

Some researchers have developed promising research surrounding intermittent fasting and the consumption of food during the day as a way to leverage the greatest metabolic advantage. According to an overview of circadian rhythms from flies to humans by *Nature* in 2002, the time of day we eat does play a large role in certain physiological processes such as hormonal secretion, coordination and sleep. The idea that meal timing is a circadian synchroniser is predominately based off animal research; but what we do know for certain is that shift work disturbs the circadian rhythms of people significantly and increases their risk of obesity, cardiovascular disease and even cancer.

Research from *Obesity* journal in 2013 shows us that consuming the majority of food during the early hours of the day is associated with lower weight and improved health. If food was available then a Palaeolithic man may have eaten breakfast, but there was a natural balance occurring between scarcity of food and abundance of food. We have rid ourselves of that balance. So for the optimal fasting schedule we could use the example for the sixteen/eight fast. This involves eating from 10 a.m. to 6 p.m. and fasting from 6 p.m. to10 a.m., or eating from 6 a.m. to 2 p.m. and fasting from 2 p.m. to 6 a.m. Remember, just because this *could* be more optimal physiologically, that doesn't mean that it's going to be optimal for you. I urge you to make the decision of when you are scheduling your fast on the grounds of logistical/social reasons over the potential metabolic benefits of fasting at a different time. But try your best to never eat large quantities of food within the last few hours of wakefulness. Especially cheese! It gives you the weirdest dreams, or is that just me?

The most frequent advice you hear regarding sleep is eight hours as a benchmark for a healthy sleep. A review of recent research at the National Sleep Foundation shows that the spectrum has widened (although eight hours not a bad place to start). Experts seem to agree that seven to nine hours is best for those aged 18–64. The amount of sleep you need depends on your genetics, age, lifestyle, activity level, your stress levels and also your ability to manage stress. If you're weight training, especially doing very heavy lifts, such as cleans, jerks, deadlifts and squats multiple times per week, you may need slightly over nine hours. Base your judgement on your sleep requirement not on the number itself, but on how a certain amount of sleep affects *you* (another variable in life useful to track in a journal). A simple way to make this judgement is to see how many hours of sleep you need to function and complete your daily tasks adequately without the use of stimulants such as caffeine (given a week or so in order to wear off tolerance).

Sleep medicine specialist Dr Robert Rosenberg warns that studies have shown too much sleep on a regular basis can increase the risk of diabetes, heart disease, stroke and death. He defines "too much" as greater than nine hours per night. (This is different for younger children and adolescence as their bodies are constantly growing.) It's important to find the sweet spot through self-experimentation and not by simply attaching oneself to anecdotal advice from friends, family or even from clinical sources as an absolute.

As we've seen, the amount of sleep needed varies from person to person, but this doesn't give you the grounds to sleep for three hours per night. Remember that sleep deprivation – although felt quickly – can worsen exponentially over time because stress is cumulative. Lack of sleep is easy to be unaware of as we're all constantly exposed to stimulation. As a consequence you may end up in a situation where you need your full mental or physical alertness but lack the ability to exert yourself as necessary, despite the misconception that you are well-rested.

If you are new to exercise, or you haven't yet adopted a regular routine around strength training or any other athletic pursuit, you will most likely need more sleep. As you break down the integrity of your muscle fibres through training your body, more sleep is required to adequately recover through the process of protein synthesis and the recovery/adaptation of your central nervous system (CNS). It is important to take care when beginning any programme which is shifting into a more active lifestyle. This is true for any programme which requires constant progressive overload and improvement.

Consistently track your sleep and its effects. For instance, a conclusion you may come to is: "When I work out three times per week (strength) at forty-five minutes per season, I'm in a caloric deficit of around 500 calories and I have examinations at university – 8.5 hours of sleep suited me best during this time." Four months later: "When I work out four times per week (cardio) and maintain calories – 7.5 hours was enough for me to get by."

A 2010 study from *The Journal of Clinical Endocrinology & Metabolism* looked at patterns of growth hormone (GH) and cortisol in relation to sleep and wakefulness. Plasma hormone levels were monitored in ten young men during baseline waking and sleeping during forty hours of wakefulness, and during sleep following deprivation. The normal nocturnal GH surge disappeared with sleep deprivation and intensified following sleep deprivation. This hormone isn't referred to as the "fountain of youth" for nothing, as it is essential to the stimulation of growth and repair of your body. Many people choose to go without sleep because they want to get more work done throughout the day. The irony of this is that those who deprive themselves out of good intention generally become the *least* productive and the least happy.

REM SLEEP

Sleep is broken down into different stages of either *rapid eye movement* (REM) or *non-rapid eye movement* (NREM) sleep. REM sleep is the term given to the two stages of sleep where eye movement occurs rapidly in random directions. During this time we experience extremely vivid or even lucid dreams. REM sleep occurs around stages four and five of sleep, right before the time you wake up. You may notice that your most vivid dreams are interrupted by the sound of your alarm. REM sleep occupies around 20-25 per cent of our sleep.

NREM Sleep

Non-rapid eye movement is sleep which, as the name suggests, has no rapid eye movement. NREM has three distinct stages. These stages are referred to as N1, N2 and N3. N1 and N2 are light sleep, which you experience during a short nap. N3 happens after several continuous hours of sleep and can be called "deep sleep".

- 6 a.m. Cortisol in the body increases dramatically
- 7.30 a.m. Melatonin secretion stops
- 9 a.m. Secretion of testosterone peaks
- 10 a.m. Alertness and productivity peaks
- 2.30 p.m. Optimal coordination
- 3.30 p.m. Our reaction times are at their best
- 5 p.m. Muscular strength and cardiovascular ability peaks
- 7 p.m. Increased blood pressure and overall temperature of the body
- 9 p.m. The release of melatonin begins again
- 10.30 p.m. Bowel urges and movement stop
- 2 a.m. Deep sleep
- 4.30 a.m. The body cools to its lowest temperature

What Time Should You Sleep?

A 1997 study from the *Journal of Psychosomatic Research* set out to find whether quality or quantity is more important for sleep. Subjects were to complete a seven-day scheme where a sleep log was used to monitor overall well-being and fatigue of the participants. The results made it clear that quality should never be neglected. Timing is very relevant to the circadian rhythm and this backs up the phrase "not all sleep is made the same". Much of the way we experience the day will be predetermined somewhat by the time we actually fall asleep. This is why aiming for a certain number of hours asleep can be pointless, when other factors can be just as important.

To function at your best and recover properly it's important to be in a relative equilibrium of REM and NREM sleep. You can increase the likelihood of this occurring by sleeping between 8 p.m.–12 a.m. Yes, some people are naturally inclined to sleep late and some earlier, but this still remains inclusive of this time bracket; it doesn't excuse staying awake until 3 a.m. This natural inclination to sleep earlier or later and likewise rise differently is referred to as your chronotype (coming from the Greek word *chrono*, meaning "time"). Your chronotype is your natural inclination to sleep at a specific time based on a multitude of genetic and environmental factors. Listen to your chronotype and become aware of it, but also respect the universal time bracket for optimum sleep and fit your schedule within it.

Research findings from the 27th annual meeting of the Associated Professional Sleep Societies suggest that sunlight, a *zeitgeber* (external factor which can affect the circadian rhythm) is one of the best antidotes for the affected chronic insomniac. The study tracked the quality of sleep for forty-nine shift workers in an office. Twenty-seven of these workers had no window and twenty-two had an abundance of natural light. The aim was to find whether exposure to natural light during the day correlated to a better quality sleep at night. The tool used to evaluate the quality of sleep was called the Pittsburgh Sleep Quality Index (PSQI). As well as this index an actigraphy (a non-invasive tool) was used to monitor the rest and activity cycles of the participants. The results showed that those exposed to sunlight did sleep better, sleeping forty-six minutes longer per night (and receiving 173 per cent more sunlight), compared to the group which had no exposure. Get some sun! Try to aim for at the very least fifteen minutes of sun exposure, although thirty to forty-five minutes is more ideal. My favourite thing to do is go on a walk in the morning, listen to an audiobook and use this time to wake up. It's a strategy

I used for one of my online clients who has trouble sleeping early and it seems to be working well.

Most people will spend the last few hours of the day on their phones and laptops. Electronic screens are designed to look like the sun. At night this light can be harmful to both the quality of your sleep and your ability to sleep. However, there is software and apps which change the lighting output of your screen in accordance to the time of day to emulate more natural light, and therefore promote ideal hormonal fluctuations in the body.

Interrupted sleep, commonly known as napping, has become a popular method of increasing productivity and decreasing stress. Naps are so effective that it has raised the question as to whether human are polyphasic sleepers by nature. The majority of mammals (85 per cent) are polyphasic – that is, they sleep more than once per day. Monophasic sleep is how most of Western cultures operate, with two distinct periods of rest and alertness. In some cultures – predominately in southern Europe – most people will sleep in the early to mid-afternoon.

This isn't about re-framing our cultural norms, and you don't necessarily have to take naps if you're getting enough sleep as it is and a monophasic lifestyle suits you. However, for some of you, your lifestyle depends on working hours that require your fullest attention at very early and/or very late hours of the day. Adopting an interrupted sleeping pattern may be the solution you need. These sleeping patterns can further be divided into three categories.

1. **Intentional nap:** Intentional naps when you're not actually tired. This type is useful when you already know you're going to have to stay up later than normal.

2. **Emergency nap:** An emergency nap is when you get tired when you least expected it (perhaps this could be because of cumulative stress catching up with you). Having a nap will allow you to re-energise and perform at your best.

3. **Habitual nap:** You shouldn't take a nap for longer than thirty minutes if you are seeking immediate cognitive and physical benefits. Brief naps (five to twenty minutes) allow an individual to reap the energetic and cognitive benefits almost immediately. As you approach the thirty-minute mark, there will be a slight sleep inertia for a brief period if you sleep any longer. However, improved performance lasts for many hours if you exceed thirty minutes.

Some tips for better sleep:

- Sleep in complete darkness.
- Maintain a regular sleeping schedule.
- See light as soon as possible in the morning.
- Stop looking at electronics before bed (or use *f.lux*).
- Use your bedroom for sleep and sex, nothing else.
- Maintain a regular sleep schedule.
- Avoid smoking and nicotine.
- Do not watch television in your bedroom.
- Sleep in a slightly cool room.
- Avoid caffeine in the afternoon/evening.
- Brush your teeth slightly earlier than normal.
- Sleep on a hard surface.

Some Stoics believed in practical practices like sleeping on the floor. Very soft beds are not the best for the health of our backs and posture. While you're asleep your body needs some sort of resistance so that your muscles become free and blood is able to circulate with greater ease. When you're sleeping on a harder surface, your lower back does not collapse as you lay on it due to the pressure from beneath. This pressure allows the lungs to inhale more oxygen more freely. Refraining from sleeping on a very soft bed can be a great way to improve some aspects of your life with little effort other than making that decision and getting used to it. Anecdotally, I found the health of my back improve greatly after backpacking in south-east Asia where beds are noticeably harder than in New Zealand.

EVENING RETROSPECTIONS

At night we must review what happened during the day, even if in the moment the act seems trivial. Evening meditation and retrospective techniques are extremely useful for examining the tasks and events which precede nightfall. The Pythagoreans (another group of philosophers from ancient Greece) practised meditations three times a day. They used evening meditative techniques as a way to improve their memory and reasoning, while Stoic teachers such as Epictetus focused more on retrospection. Seneca depicts evening retrospections as a practice to be taken as seriously as an appearance before court. For a very brief moment in our day we must be completely honest with ourselves and express our observations, improvements or lack thereof, and most critically, the reasons *why* this occurred.

Whether you are tracking your progress in self-control for sugary foods, the frequency you're attending the gym, or any task, understand that anything in the past is out of your control. Anything that is out of control should not be approached with a perspective of what could have been done; we look at these past events with indifference. Ask yourself how you could improve moving forward; rephrase *could* into what *will* you do from now on.

If you are asking yourself how your nutrition was today, and you realise you ate too much chocolate, instead of feeling disappointed and pondering on the negative association that eating chocolate has brought to your progress, try this instead. Look at what came before you ate the chocolate: the environment, the mindset. Ask yourself what set the stage for this momentary vice to surface. Look at every pattern to see if there's anything you can do differently to create a more virtuous outcome in the future. Think how you can apply your questioning of "what am I doing now?" to these future situations where you do have control over your decisions. Evening meditations will help you sleep as you rid yourself of wavering thoughts.

Insomnia is the habitual inability to sleep because of constant overthinking. Retrospections take care of this. As Epictetus explains: "Allow not sleep to close your wearied eyes until you have reckoned up each daytime deed: 'Where did I go wrong? What did I do? And what duty's left undone?' From first to last review your acts and then reprove yourself for wretched [or cowardly] acts, but rejoice in those done well."

I spoke earlier about turning off your electronics before bed, as with brushing your teeth earlier, to signal to yourself that eating and wakefulness is over. Use your evening meditations as a cue to transition from wakefulness into rest.

I will use the example of "Max" as someone who is trying to eat healthy and quit smoking cigarettes.

Max writes in his journal: "What evils have you cured yourself of today?"

He answers the question: "Today I was offered Coca-Cola and I turned down the offer twice. The second time the temptation was so strong but I managed to fight through the urge and resisted my own desire! I also ate five servings of fruits and vegetables and was able to hold my fasting window for sixteen hours."

"In what sense are you better?"

"I have never squatted over 100 kg, but today I set a personal record and squatted 102.5 kg. Never in my life did I think this would have been possible. I'm proud and I'm looking forward to future challenges."

"What did you omit today?"

"I didn't finish the rest of my workout after I broke my personal record. I was satisfied with this accomplishment, so much so that I could not concentrate on the rest of my workout.

I should be proud that I accomplished something, but not let this derail me from what I had planned to do. Self-control and discipline aren't made out of accomplishment, they are defined through consistency."

"What vices have you fought?"

"I have fought my urge to smoke the usual six cigarettes, although I still smoked two. I made progress but I am clearly still dependent as I still wake up craving nicotine within minutes. I know that normalcy will only come through resisting this urge, but progress is progress and for this, I am grateful."

Your evening meditations don't have to be this long, or this short, as long as you are honest.

If you are more artistic, sketching can be a great addition, but not always a good replacement. For the more Socratic folk a voice recording will suffice. There will be days where you may write more than others, some days you may have much to ponder on but little to write, and others where you are at the store buying extra paper. If you can't think of anything to write, then write that you're stuck for words – just write *something!*

I hope by reading through the examples above you can see just how much of a difference this could do for your accountability over time. Imagine looking back through years of entries. Do not fear being critical of yourself, as you are your most acclaimed and highest critic. Don't let this become an outlet for only the negative, and likewise do not frame your retrospections as explicitly positive. Prevent bias and denial from taking your words; allow your honesty and indifference to frame nothing but rational honesty with the self and constant progression towards virtue. Musonius tells us is that if we are practising each virtue we must move forward in the lessons these practices teaches us; if we don't move forward, there is no point in learning about them in the first place.

APPROPRIATING REST

Zeno was asked why he relaxed when he was at a dinner party and his reply was that, "Lupins too are bitter, but when they are soaked they become sweet." In *Apophthegms*, the second book by Hecato (a Stoic philosopher from Rhodes), Zeno's habits have become almost a proverb: "More temperate than Zeno the philosopher." In *Men Transported*, Greek poet Posidippus says: "So that for ten whole days he did appear more temperate than Zeno's self." However, this doesn't mean that rest isn't necessary and that indulging doesn't have its place.

Stoic philosopher Cato the Younger used to rejuvenate his mind with red wine. We know that Cato particularly loved wine that came from grapes which received the most sunshine, testimony to his love of the drink. As I said, moderate alcoholic consumption is not forbidden to Stoics. Seneca tells us that men ought to have relaxation, as those who rest after labour rise up better than before. Seneca gives an example of crop fields, telling us that we mustn't force crops from rich fields as heavy crops in an "unbroken course" exhaust the fertility of the soil, just as our minds can become injured through labour which never ceases.

Seneca continues: "Our ancestors, too, forbade any new motion to be made in the Senate after the tenth hour. Soldiers divide their watches, and those who have just returned from active service are allowed to sleep the whole night undisturbed." We account for breaks, eating the occasional slice of cake, watching television – but doesn't this distract us from the virtue we must attend to? There's a pitfall in restriction. We should accept that things are desirable but *aren't* necessary, rather than rejecting that things *are* desirable.

PART SEVEN:
VOLUNTARY DISCOMFORT

"Provide things relating to the body no further than mere use; as meat, drink, clothing, house, family. But strike off and reject everything relating to show and delicacy."

-Epictetus

THE PARADOX OF PAIN AND PLEASURE

"If a person is struck by an arrow, is it painful? If the person is struck by a second arrow, is it even more painful?"

The Buddhist parable of "The Arrow" gives the perfect introduction to a discussion of pain. Pain, injury and physical distress: these are all experiences which are usually associated with suffering and misery. Whether this pain is emotional or physical, it can feel as if a poisoned arrow has pierced the skin.

The reaction for the ordinary person when pierced by a "poisoned arrow" is to seek the opposite. Pleasure is sought after pain in order to comfort ourselves. But we must question whether it is it right to seek out aversion. To detach yourself from pain and only perceive it as a physical sensation will free your mind from distress and allow you to deal with it in a manner where it becomes an experience undefined by external anguish and suffering. To allow your mind to manifest the sensation as *both* physical and mental is the mistake most make.

Yes, I understand that clearly this is easier said than done. Buddhism tells us that we cannot always control the first arrow. However, the second arrow is our reaction to the first. This second arrow is optional. Both Marcus Aurelius and Epictetus tell us that our body is not actually fully in our control. Marcus Aurelius says, "Our inevitable experience of pain through injury and disease are for the most part out of our control." We can never be free of pain because tearing your hamstring on a deadlift *hurts*, we all know this. Pain cannot be avoided, but what we can master is the art of being free from distress brought on by the pain. Pain becomes not just a simple sensation, but the failure to avoid what we mistake as "bad".

WHAT EXACTLY IS PAIN?

The internet and the age of self-diagnosis allows us to overreact to minor pain or injury. "I have a headache and this website tells me a headache is the symptom of X cause" – this scenario is not uncommon. It is difficult to analyse a human experience such as pain, as the experience itself is subjective. This subjectivity is not exclusive to the psychology of the individual but also to the sensitivity of nerve endings. An extreme example would be a genetic disorder such as congenital analgesia (CIP), where no pain is felt at all. For these individuals Stoicism would come naturally. All jokes aside, let's explore the physiological process behind pain.

Pain begins with the activation of receptors called nociceptors; these nociceptors are distributed throughout all of our muscular tissue, our joints, ligaments, spine and fascia (connective tissues). If we were to examine a nociceptor, we would see individual nerve endings which hold one purpose

– to identify tissue damage via chemical singling which then travels to the brain.

When tissue is damaged from exercising, nutrients and fluids then flow into the muscle in order to repair damage. Inflammation is a well-known consequence of this process – many have the perception that inflammation is somehow bad, but inflammation is your body working as it should. Inflammation means your body is notifying you that attention is required in a certain area. This doesn't mean you shouldn't respond appropriately through means of icing an injured area. Instead, simply be grateful that your body is functioning as it should.

Delayed onset muscle soreness (DOMS) is the well-known experience which every regular gym goer will endure in the days following a gruelling workout. This pain is also referred to as "muscle fever". Depending on the intensity of the exercise and muscles exercised, this pain can last for several days (it's usually most noticeable in the twenty-four to seventy-two hours following exercise). You may also experience pain directly after or even during exercise, but this shouldn't be confused with DOMS. Acute muscle soreness refers to pain in the moments immediately following exercise. Delayed onset muscle soreness helps prevent damage to the muscles. Your muscle tissue experiences micro traumas, which causes the pain. These micro traumas must repair in order to improve the integrity, size and strength of the muscle in order to adapt to the progressive stress your body expects in future workouts. This is the basis for progressive overload.

Lactic acid is not actually fully responsible for the soreness; rather it is a by-product of it. The belief that lactic acid causes DOMS is an outdated idea. The eccentric part of a resistance based movement is the cause of most trauma. When your muscles are in an eccentric movement pattern with some type of resistance they are lengthening. It is at this point that the fibres of a muscle are much more vulnerable to being damaged. There has also been recent speculation that the pain following exercise is not specifically caused by damage to the tissue, but due to damage of the fascia (connective tissue).

'SOLUTIONS' TO PAIN?

> "Let the leading and ruling part of your soul stand unmoved by the stirrings of the flesh, whether gentle or rude. Let it not commingle with them, but keep itself apart, and confine these passions to their proper bodily parts; and if they rise into the soul by any sympathy with the body to which it is united, then we must not attempt to resist the sensation, seeing that it is of our nature; but let not the soul, for its part, add thereto the conception that the sensation is good or bad."

> – Marcus Aurelius

It's often assumed that over-the-counter (OTC) medication is relatively risk-free on the grounds that it requires no prescription. Even safe medication like paracetamol (known as acetaminophen or APAP) can cause kidney or liver failure if consumed on an empty stomach at twice the recommended dose. The fact that in many places it's legal to advertise medication on TV gives the dangerous impression that every problem can be solved by self-medicating.

With the uncomfortable pain that comes after exercise there will of course be many solutions to the issue through supplementation. There have been studies showing that caffeine effectively reduces pain post-exercise. A study in 2007 from the *Journal of Pain* showed a moderate intake of caffeine (two cups of coffee) can reduce pain post-workout by nearly 50 per cent. According to pain researcher Patrick J. O'Connor:

"A lot of times what people use for muscle pain is aspirin or ibuprofen, but caffeine seems to work better than those drugs, at least among women whose daily caffeine consumption is low." Another study in 2003 from the *Journal of Pain* has shown that caffeine can reduce pain during moderately intense training. What is important to note is that caffeine tolerance is relevant to how effective caffeine will be in treating pain.

Omega-3 fats are known for health benefits. The form of omega-3 fats come in Docosahexaenoic acid (DHA), eicosapentaenoic acid (EPA) and alpha-linoleic acid (ALA). ALA is found in certain seeds, nuts and some dairy, whereas EPA and DHA (which ALA can convert to) is found in fatty fish such as salmon. Omega-3 is most commonly advertised as fish oil. Fish oil was compared in a study to non-steroidal anti-inflammatory drugs (NSAID), commonly known as ibuprofen. In 2004, over several months, 250 patients with back or neck pain took 1200mg per day of omega-3 EFAs (an average dose) and the results showed that over half (59 per cent) of participants stopped using NSAIDs for the pain; while most (88 per cent) said they would continue to use the fish oil. What is most noteworthy is that there were no side effects.

Fatty acids omega-3 and omega-6 are identical to the chemist, but to our cells they are not. An important part of health and fat loss is to rid the body of inflammation; this reduction allows cells to better communicate. People eat far too much omega-6 because of the typical Western diet, while omega-3 fatty acids are what most people's bodies are lacking, hence the popularity of the supplement. A major European randomised clinical trial has shown us that fish oil does work, it protects the heart and has various other benefits including reducing depression, anxiety, bowel inflammation and even arthritis. When supplementing, we're looking for EPA and DHA. There is no set dose for EPA and DHA because different individuals require different quantities. For reference, ALA (alpha-linoleic acid) is the type of omega-3 found in plant-based sources such as chia seed and flaxseed.

From researching various sources I think a good place to start is between 1-3 g of the active compounds. For the best "type" of omega-3 consider krill as your first option. Both the EPA and DHA in krill oil are more bioavailable because of phospholipids. Krill also has astaxanthin which protects DHA in our cell membranes. A 2011 study from *Lipids* journal shows that the metabolic effects of krill oil are essentially similar to those of fish oil but at lower dose of EPA and DHA.

While on the topic of supplements, although they are not required if you have a healthy diet, there are certain means of supplementation which can be extremely beneficial. I've already mentioned fish oil but there are others, according to a "scorecard" of supplements published by Harvard University Medical School in 2012. These include fibre, selenium and the "three Bs" – vitamin B6 (pyridoxine), folate (folic acid, which is synthetic) and B12 (cobalamin).

10 adaptogenic herbs for reducing inflammation/pain:
- Valerian (*Valeriana officinalis*)
- Devil's claw (*Harpagophytum procumbens*)
- White willow (*Salix alba*)
- Turmeric (*Curcuma longa*)
- Bromelain (stems of pineapple)
- Sour cherry (*Prunus cerasus*)
- Ginger (*Zingiber officinale*)
- Eucommia *(Eucommia ulmoides)*
- *Boswellia serrata (Olibaum Indicum)*
- Guggul *(Commiphora wightii)*

These herbs are a great addition to a balanced diet, but of course are not required. With your current understanding of Stoicism you may question whether it is truly appropriate to use NSAIDs supplements. The truth lies in how you view the pleasure you are receiving from these solutions. Less so the adaptogenic herbs as they pose little risk for abuse and harm (but be aware some can have side effects). You can use an external source to alleviate your pain but do not let that become your pleasure and source of comfort. In *Discourses*, Epictetus wrote: "I have a headache. Well, do not say 'Alas! I have an earache.' Do not say 'Alas!' And I am not saying that it is not permissible to groan, only do not groan in the centre of your being." What Epictetus is saying is that Stoicism isn't about *repressing* your responses to external influences. Pain is a natural experience. It's impossible to never express your anguish as this is unnatural and restrictive; the point is to not centre your being around the "alas".

If we take a squat for example, in the coming days where DOMS is felt, it's not the pain of your legs that should make you happy or unhappy. Your expression of your discomfort is permissible, but this experience shouldn't be one that you see as evil. Your "alas" is a recognition of what is real, not what you fear it to become. Although it may seem senseless to overanalyse the pain from the day after squats, swimming, gymnastics or martial arts – which is nothing more than a nuisance in comparison tearing a muscle or breaking a bone – there's still merit in this. However, doing this consistently will allow you to build resistance to the larger pains which may happen in your life.

American psychologist Richard Solomon came up with a remarkable theory called the opponent-process theory of acquired motivation, in which he explores the paradoxical nature of pain and pleasure. Mr Solomon analysed the opposing experiences of pleasure and pain and argued that either can turn into a dependency based on the premise that one invokes the opposite experience, given the appropriate circumstances. The opponent-process theory has shown us that dependency is due to the combination of pleasure and emotional responses which come with the withdrawal of a substance an individual is dependent on. During the beginning of use, pleasure is high and withdrawal is low. As the pleasure and dependency increases with use, the withdrawal symptoms increase and worsen, and this provokes a behaviour where something is no longer pleasurable yet still remains persuasive enough to the individual to invoke persistent and consistent desire for more.

To better understand this, think about drug addicts who commit violent crimes against their nature, throwing out morals they used to pride themselves on in order to obtain a substance which actually brings them no pleasure. It is the same for food. Although an individual may not necessarily commit violent crimes for a burger (although it's not unheard of), money, time and effort is spent in order to acquire something which objectively serves no real pleasure. It's a horrible cycle.

Mr Solomon's idea of the interchange between pleasure and pain is similar to the pleasure zones of food we previously covered. An individual who is addicted to sugar may very well have simply been an occasional user – as with a social smoker or a social drinker – before it became a visible concern. The difference between the attached and the detached individual is that the dependent person experiences pain in absence of the pleasure. Over time when there is scarcity of the pleasure, they may have felt a longing for the pleasurable experience for multiple reasons – boredom, melancholy, or anything else. This pleasure is desired as the freedom of access disappears. Gradually this forms into a dependent association of happiness with the intake of certain foods or substances. Over time, this reinforces a stronger relationship between their perception of what makes them happy and what is actually causing their pain. We've already covered this and so there's no need to elaborate. What I would like to speak about now is the inverse relationship between pain and pleasure.

Exercise-induced euphoria is the term used to describe the feeling that comes from exercise, especially during bouts of high intensity. The well-known "runners' high" is an example of the link between pain and pleasure. In this instance, the pain and discomfort of endurance running becomes a pleasurable, or even euphoric, experience, resembling a high. According to Mr Solomon this activity begins to become associated with greater pain for greater pleasure. The longer the run or the more intense the workout, the greater the pleasure that will result for the individual. This isn't to necessarily claim that pain to pleasure is more desirable than pleasure to pain. Excluding masochism, the relationship between pain and pleasure is what we seem to be lacking as a society. Pain becomes a pleasure; it doesn't transcend it. Professor William B. Irvine reintroduces the ancient idea of *hedonic adaptation*, which was well-established through the work of psychologists Shane Frederick and George Lowenstein. Hedonic adaptation is the idea that external happiness doesn't stay for long. If you magically received the body of your dreams, all the money in the world and everything you had ever dreamed of, you wouldn't necessarily be as happy as you might expect to be. In some instances, you might find more pain in the immediate pleasure you were abruptly exposed to.

As an example, one of my worst nightmares is winning the lottery. This may seem absolutely absurd, but I know that if I won the lottery in my younger years it may take away from the hustle and the investment which is so important to put towards yourself as you improve as a young man. The individual who wins the lottery or magically gets the body of their dreams would resort back to the baseline very quickly. Their consciousness has no time to adapt to such a large shift in their environment. They didn't go through the frequent tests of willpower and discomfort to obtain their desires.

We can compare this example to the shortcuts people will take to achieve health and beauty through the use of anabolic androgens (steroids). Ask yourself who is going to be more satisfied with a six-pack – the one who goes about it the more difficult way (ten years of hard work) or the individual who achieves the same in one year through the use of androgens? I don't mean disrespect to those who choose to use androgens, but doing so contradicts the very essence of what being a healthy person means, physiologically and psychologically.

Any stimulus, whether physical or emotional, kick-starts the opponent processes. This doesn't necessarily mean that you must go out of your way to avoid what is pleasurable. The answer is to moderate your frequency of exposure to pleasurable stimuli and intentionally increase exposure to moderate pain and discomfort in order to come to a therapeutic equilibrium between both opponent forces. We can build pressure by intentionally exposing ourselves to various stresses. Stresses (intermittent fasting, plain food, cold showers) are short-lived. Your nervous system builds a tolerance to the pressure in order to defend, counter and adapt your tolerance. This is represented well in the progressive overloading methods of athletic performance. By increasing the overload of stress exposures we aren't just building a tolerance to the experience, we are building up the tone of pleasurable emotions.

> "Anger is that which goes beyond reason and carries her away with it: wherefore the first confusion of a man's mind when struck by what seems an injury is no more anger than the apparent injury itself: it is the subsequent mad rush, which not only receives the impression of the apparent injury, but acts upon it as true, that is anger, being an exciting of the mind to revenge, which proceeds from choice and deliberate resolve."

> – Seneca

Chrysippus explains the disobedience of reason with the metaphor of a runner who is moving too quickly and cannot stop his own legs at will. This scenario presents an opportunity to fulfil the craving the ego has for its desires and continues to run even if the end consequence is twisting of the ankle.

A true sage has no appetites or desires, however they do have wishes. They wish to improve and progress, despite having no appetites. Perfect wisdom is to be detached from irrational emotional and this point itself is one of Stoicism's largest contributions to modern philosophy.

DISLOCATED TRUTHS

> "But neither a bull nor a noble-spirited man comes to be what he is all at once; he must undertake hard winter training, and prepare himself, and not propel himself rashly into what is not appropriate to him."
>
> – Epictetus

Before I begin the discussion on how to successfully embrace discomforts in your life I have some interesting ideas for you to think about. One profound idea to get your head around, which I didn't previously mention, is that fasting is an example of a *dislocated truth*. So many cultures, traditions, philosophies and religions have elements of intermittent fasting – yet they were unaware of each other's existence. If there's some folk tale from Latvia telling the same story as one in Rome, then obviously there's some distinct truth being brought to light about human nature. Perhaps it is a coincidence, but the more these coincidences occur, the higher the chance of universal truth.

Carl Jung expressed a similar concept which he called *collective unconsciousness*. We can use the classic hero role as an example. The moment you sit down to watch a film (or stand up if you've been reading carefully) the character's archetypes are revealed and almost instantaneously established in the collective unconscious of the audience. This could also be applied to social interactions and first impressions. The example of the hero was true in ancient times in plays, so this shows it is true to our nature.

Perhaps I'm over-poeticising the very mundane details of everyday life, but what else are we going to do? I'm kidding of course…the point being that over-poeticising the mundane is *exactly* the point. Think about it – who are you to distinguish mundane from extraordinary at first glance? The proof in the worth of the thing may be seen right away and thus it is extraordinary, or it may take time it to reveal itself and so it is still extraordinary. It's foolish to think that small discomforts or comforts don't collectively accumulate to wider and more profound implications in life.

Zeno says, "Well-being is attained by little and little, but nevertheless is no little thing itself." From this thought came the famous book *The Slight Edge*, by Jeff Olson, among others; but Zeno's economic summary is all you need. Never underestimate the smallest moments in life; they define you as a person. Why are we told to make our beds as children, brush our teeth, save one extra dollar coin per day? This is how success is universally cultivated.

EMBRACE DISCOMFORT

Seneca warns us: "It is in times of security that the spirit should be preparing itself for difficult times; while fortune is bestowing favours on it is then is the time for it to be strengthened against her rebuffs." In plain English this means that comfort is found in discomfort. Seneca rejoiced in having little. He suggests that you must get away from the comfort of your home and your bed and everything you attach yourself to, and put yourself head first into "want" and then, as he says, you'll ask yourself, "Is this what I used to dread?"

Comfort is a horrible sort of slavery to oneself, always in fear of having something which brings you comfort being taken away. The more you can practise this discomfort at any given opportunity, the more you lessen the chance of being deeply disrupted by losses – which *will* come sooner or later.

The Stoics don't embrace the discomforts of cold or

sleeping on a hard floor out of masochism; rather the Stoics advocate for the deliberate use of discomfort to raise the appreciation for what they currently have. As explained by the process-opponent theory, by deliberately accepting an experience that invokes discomfort we "immunise" ourselves to future discomfort that we don't have full control over.

Any practice which defies social norms, such as fasting, will attract criticism both from the external and from your own internal reflections. Ignore this narrative through understanding the power of defying the norm. As William Irvine explains, "By practicing Stoic self-denial techniques over a long period, Stoics can transform themselves into individuals remarkable for their courage and self-control." Irvine is simply telling us that through these feats of discomfort, a Stoic will be able to accomplish what no normal man can.

Similar to the warning Musonius gives us on the overconsumption of meat and its digestive and cognitive disadvantage, we can see scientific parallels between these discomforts and our biology. Discomforts mimic what our evolutionary programming "expects" our day-to-day life to involve. Some of the smallest, seemingly unimportant moments of life are the seeds which sprout larger change. We can see this in nature – a plant which is troubled by the force of wind grows stronger and more resilient to future storms. If you are unable to withstand a slight discomfort for a brief period of the day, how will you cope with greater adversity when placed in a vulnerable, uncomfortable situation?

Epictetus questioned who would have power over himself if he was exposed to discomfort: "Philip or Alexander, or Perdiccas, or the Persian king? How should they have it? For he that can be subjected by man must, long before, let himself be subjected to things. He, therefore, whom neither pleasure nor pain, nor fame nor riches, can get the better of, and who is able, whenever he thinks fit, to spit his whole body into his tormentor's face and depart from life, whose slave can he ever be? To whom is he the subject?"

You don't necessarily have to partake in multiple discomforts at once. I think it's better to focus one or two and really explore and master their complexity. There may be a certain point where the paradox of pain and pleasure comes into effect and you are desensitised to the discomfort. When this inevitably occurs, as it would in the gym, find a way to progressively overload the discomfort. This doesn't necessarily mean exposing yourself to harsher conditions (although this may be a viable option with certain discomforts). An example would be extending your fasting window from sixteen hours to twenty hours, or eating plain oats and subtracting the typical quantity of sauce and flavouring you use. Remember to cycle your discomforts, but do so only when you have mastered one.

Ten voluntary discomforts:

- Cold therapy (showers, fewer clothes, drinking cold water)
- Simple food (plain rice, potato, oatmeal, vegetables)
- Prolonged fasting windows
- Sleeping on the floor and/or no pillow
- Challenging yoga positions
- Spending time in hot weather
- Drinking only water
- Zero sugar
- Attempting to surpass previous records (running, weights, swimming)
- Standing instead of sitting, barefoot running/walking

Seneca explains to us again and again that in life, bad things will inevitably happen. He used negative visualisation as a tool to help bring forth greater gratitude for his current circumstances. Poverty is the greatest means to determine whether you are content with what you truly need and desire, and I could not agree more. Think about your life right now: if everything were to be taken away, would you still be as elated as you are now? If you were elated, happy, driven, motivated, at any point in the last week, would this temporary feeling regress back to a mean of suffering which the external world had formed a crutch for?

I want to repeat this, because I think this is an extremely important question to ask yourself on a regular basis. This relates back to our discussion on *prosochē* and contemplation. Ask yourself, "What are you doing?" and "Why are you doing it?" I want you to verbalise this and ask yourself the following question:

"If I had nothing, would I still be happy?"

Well...would you?

Perhaps this answer changes from time to time and your answer is, "It depends," with two possible answers:

1. In some circumstances you may feel content knowing that you would be just as elated, whatever your environment.

2. At other times your peace of mind may depend on material and external things.

Ask yourself this question regularly so you can determine what is of vice or virtue, and gravitate towards the good option.

ASCETICISM

Asceticism simply means "exercises" or "training". A central practice of asceticism is denying all universal pleasure for spiritual or religious reasons. Asceticism is symbolic of a frugal lifestyle and abstinence from material possessions, and it is diametrically opposed to Hedonism. According to Vincent Wimbush and Richard Valantasis, who edited the book *Asceticism* in 2002, asceticism can be classified into two distinct types:

1. *Natural asceticism* is a frugal and simplistic lifestyle. What is important to remember is that this minimal lifestyle is exclusive of exposing oneself voluntarily to pain (this could perhaps be aligned to the modern "minimalist").

2. *Unnatural asceticism* is characterised by the practices which involve the body's mortification and pain. An example could be walking through snow in bare feet or sleeping on a bed of nails (ouch!).

Friedrich Nietzsche held an interesting perceptive on asceticism which can be found in his book *On the Genealogy of Morals,* specifically in his third essay, "What Do Ascetic Ideals Mean?" In this essay Nietzsche discusses what he sees as the ascetic ideal and how this ideal plays an important role in the formulation of morality relative to the history of the "will". Nietzsche described the paradoxical interchange between pain and pleasure (which I covered earlier in this chapter through the work of Richard Solomon) as an action which may be of value to life itself. Through these ascetic acts you can surpass your fear and desire to run from the uncomfortable, and so remain masterful over the self.

Stoicism is frequently, but mistakenly, seen as an ascetic philosophy. Unlike ascetics, Stoicism didn't advocate suffering for its own sake – instead it focuses on *apatheia*, or equanimity. There's nothing bad about asceticism, but Stoicism doesn't pursue asceticism as the goal itself – it's not the vessel through which mastery is obtained. As Epictetus said: "Look at me, I have no house or city, property or slave: I sleep on the ground, I have no wife or children, no miserable palace, but only earth and sky and one poor cloak. Yet what do I lack? Am I not quit of pain and fear, am I not free?"

The justification for asceticism is based on goals, in the pursuit of specific religions and spiritual doctrines, which are often seen as being impeded by submitting to pleasure, stimulation and delight. Stoics, on the other hand, focus on being indifferent to pleasure and pain, as a tool to living in accord with nature.

impulses from nerve endings which are sent to the brain. This is likely where the "euphoric" and happy feelings post-cold shower come from. Through being exposed to cold temperatures, your body prevents potential bruising of an injured area and also clears the build-up of waste and fluid. Even if you're not injured, every time you work out you are inflicting minor damage on your muscular tissue (so technically you are injured), meaning you need to recover.

Theoretically, exposing yourself to cold on a regular basis is helping you recover quicker, which then potentially will help you progress that little bit faster. Cold temperatures are also known to numb the nerve endings in your body, which after an intense workout, or a minor injury, is a useful way to minimise pain as well as reduce swelling.

Immunity, Performance and Fat Loss

In a 2014 scientific review from the *North American Journal of Medical Sciences* on the evidence-based effects of hydrotherapy on various systems of the body, it was found that hydrotherapy can improve the overall management of pain, immunity and other diseases such as anorectal disorders, fatigue, anxiety, obesity, hypercholesterolemia, hyperthermia and labour.

The more we learn about the human body, the more we understand that much of the common advice of keeping warm and eating breakfast is simply false. Newly popularised figures such as Wim Hof (a Dutch daredevil known as "the iceman", who is able to withstand long periods of extreme cold) have certainly increased the rejection of these dogmatic ideas and fundamentally challenged some of our assumptions about what the human body is capable of.

The reason that cold showers increase your immunity to disease is because your body has an automatic reaction to cold temperatures. When cold water hits your skin your body quickly regulates your core temperature. This automatic response *increases* your metabolism and your immune system is activated.

With this rapid activation the body is then flooded with white blood cells. This release strengthens your ability to fight off disease when your immunity is compromised in the future.

A 1999 study from the *Journal of Applied Physiology* and a 1998 study from the *Journal of Interferon & Cytokine Research* found that winter swimmers have higher counts of white blood cells; these included T-lymphocytes and natural killer cells which help kill viruses and tumours. A 40 per cent decrease in incidents of respiratory tract infections was also noted. Both eleuthero *(Eleutherococcus senticosus) and* ashwagandha *(Withania somnifera)* – two of my adaptogenic herb recommendations for cortisol reduction – are also widely acknowledged to increase maximum oxygen capacity, or VO2 max. High level athletes are always trying to find ways to increase their VO2 max; this is why you'll hear stories of athletes moving to Denver, Colorado or Kathmandu, Nepal to train at higher altitudes. I've also seen athletes at my gym wear an oxygen restricting mask to mimic high-altitude conditions. A 2011 study from the *PLoS One* journal shows us that cold water does indeed improve people's VO2 max.

Mitochondria are parts of a eukaryote cell. They are known as the powerhouse of the body and their main job is the conversation of energy. Mitochondria use glucose and store it in their chemical bonds in order to make adenosine triphosphate (ATP). This process is called *cellular respiration.* ATP serves as the primary currency of the cell – you could think of it as the body's battery. It's used for many reasons, including moving substances across cell membranes and supplying energy for muscular contraction. Since mitochondria give us the ability to use oxygen for cellular energy, the more we have the more aerobic potential we have.

According to a 2014 study from *Medicine & Science in Sports & Exercise*, the PPARGC1A gene is activated when we are exposed to cold water, which creates more mitochondria in the muscle. This study had nine active males perform thirty minutes of non-stop running at 70 per cent of their maximum aerobic capacity followed by running at 100 per cent aerobic velocity until "failure". Afterwards they were asked to immerse one leg in cold water at 50°F (10°C) for fifteen minutes, three times per week for four weeks in total. The other leg served as the control and the result showed that there was a significant increase in the number of mitochondria in the muscular tissue of the leg exposed to cold water. In a 2011 study from *PLoS ONE,* another nine well-trained runners were told to run on a treadmill in order to prove muscular damage. Various cold therapy methods were used to test which would be more effective. The result was that the entire body emerged in cold water was more effective post-run (twenty-four to forty-eight hours) with a 20 per cent increase in speed and power for an additional two days.

The lymphatic system is your body's way of removing waste from your cells. Waste is removed at a faster rate by exposure to the cold. What this means is that there will be fewer bacteria and overall unwelcome guests in your body. As well as an increase in immunity, when the lymphatic system is cleared there is a unique benefit – all cells in your body are cleared. As stressful as the brief moments under extreme cold feel, your glutathione levels increase and uric acid levels decrease. Both glutathione and uric acid levels increase are closely linked to stress levels which cold showers alleviate. Improved circulation means that more blood is able to make it to your organs to keep them warm and at appropriate temperatures. When the circulatory system is activated and stimulated by increased blood flow this means overall cardiovascular health will improve (just to a lesser extent than most exercise).

There has also been some speculation about the effects cold therapy has on fat loss. We can see there is some substance to this, based on the similarity cold showers have to exercise – or more specifically, the relationship cold water has on brown fat and white fat.

Brown fat is comprised of small lipids or fat droplets which contain a large quantity of mitochondria. Iron gives this type of fat the brown colour. Brown fat is predominantly found around the upper back and its purpose is to help us warm our body through burning energy. We can, for simplicity's sake, view this fat as being useful as it can aid us in burning more calories. A 2009 study from the *New England Journal of Medicine* looked at the importance of brown adipose tissue in human adults. When subjects were exposed to cold temperatures brown fat was activated in 96 per cent of participants (twenty-three out of twenty-four). This means that for the individuals in the study an extra nine pounds per year could be lost with a consistent practice.

Brown fat is formed as we exercise and burn energy. During this time white fat is able to be converted into brown fat. There are various other variables which affect the level and production of brown fat, including the quantity and quality of your sleep, which is responsible for the body's production of melatonin. As cold therapy works in a similar fashion to exercise, cold exposure also increases the amount of brown fat in our bodies.

White fat is very different to brown. There are fewer blood vessels. It is made up of multiple small lipids or droplets with much fewer mitochondria. White fat gives our organs a cushion to lay on as we interact with the external world. White fat acts as a thermal insulator. Insulin, cortisol, adrenaline sensitivity and levels are directly influenced by the receptors in white fat is comprised of. By drinking cold water your metabolic rate is quickly increased; this is because your body must accommodate itself to the significant change in temperature. Having your skin exposed to water in the form of a shower or bath may actually help us burn more fat. Now it must be noted that it's not a replacement for exercise, and neither is this specific benefit extremely significant in itself.

Because brown fat is the type that actually burns energy instead of storing it, it's much more similar to a muscle rather than what one may typically define as fat. Any type of cold will activate this, as it simply comes down to burning more energy.

What this means for your efforts is that cold showers aren't the only method of gaining a similar benefit.

Try doing the following to get benefits out of cold temperatures:

- Drink cold water with ice.
- Use an ice pack on sore areas (specifically on the upper back/back of the neck).
- Take cold baths.
- Wear less clothing in winter.
- Walk in bare feet.

PASSIVE INCOME

Many economists will tell you that having one main stream of income, along with multiple streams of passive income, secures the accumulation of wealth. Of course this is debatable, but take this as a truth for the following analogy. We can view the right approach to your fat loss and health through a similar concept. Your efforts should come mainly from eating healthy, exercising too, but also other means such as cold immersion. Think of cold therapy as passive income to your full-time job (nutrition) and your part-time job (exercise).

ON SEXUAL PLEASURE

"The difference here between the Epicurean and our own school is this: our wise man feels his troubles but overcomes them, while their wise man does not even feel them. We share with them the belief that the wise man is content with himself."

– Seneca

In today's world there is a new movement beginning to surface, which contradicts the recently sexually liberated nature of contemporary Western culture. This next section is not an attack on this liberation. Abstaining from sexual release as a means to improve your productivity, happiness and overall quality of life is becoming popularised through movements on internet forums, especially Reddit and YouTube. To my knowledge, the idea of abstinence was originally made mainstream by author Napoleon Hill in his economics book *Think and Grow Rich*; but it is an ancient concept. Hill explains that one of his keys to riches is "sexual transmutation", which entails using your sexual energy and transmuting it into the creative sphere of your life, henceforth becoming a more productive individual who, as the title proclaims, thinks and grows richer.

Antisthenes (444–365 BC) was one of the founders of the Cynic school of philosophy and a pupil of Socrates. He was famous for his hostility to all forms of *hedone* (pleasure), particularly sexual. He is reported as saying things such as, "I'd rather be mad than feel pleasure." Diogenes of Sinope (404-323 BC) was a man who through the words of Plato (allegedly) was described as "Socrates gone mad", known best for taking Cynicism to its logical extremes, eating raw meat and sleeping in a tub. He was exiled from Sinope for disfiguring currency and later came to Athens where he met Antisthenes, eager to become one of his students. Antisthenes refused. Through Diogenes' persistence Antisthenes clearly realised his worth and accepted him as his pupil. Diogenes became another prominent figure in the foundation of Cynic philosophy. To Antisthenes, Diogenes of Sinope and their fellow Cynics, their definition of being rich was simply having no more than one needs. This was not a figure of speech; this was their ideal. The rejection of all which one has that is unnecessary was their belief.

Diogenes owned a cup which he used for eating, but as depicted in a beautiful painting, he threw away the cup after he saw a boy drinking out of his hands. Diogenes Laërtius (a different Diogenes) recounted the story: "One day, observing a child drinking out of his hands, he cast away the cup from his wallet with the words, 'A child has beaten me in plainness of living'." As Massimo Pigliucci pointed out, the relationship of the Stoic to the Cynic is similar to that of an everyday Buddhist to a Buddhist monk. Hence why the Cynics were one of the few schools the Stoics didn't actively critique and argue against.

Sexual habits have the potential to be just as degenerative as overeating, consuming excess alcohol and other pleasure-based stimuli, perhaps with less potential for long-term abuse – but the risk factor is clear. The liberation of human sexuality has led to an exponential rise to pornography as it was introduced following the industrial revolution.

Humans are the only creatures that treat sex as a recreational act, more correctly, one of abuse. It's true that sexual activity among youth in many countries has begun to decline, but my claim on the abundance of recreational sexual activity is inclusive of the self (masturbation), and if this is taken into consideration the point is again solidified even further. This is not to say that other species in the animal kingdom don't have sex with the absolute purpose of pleasure; but every animal approaches sex with moderation, even if the purpose is not exclusive to procreation.

I've made it very clear through discussing one's relationship to food and other pleasures with potential for harm, that irrational value judgements can bring dangers. With this in mind we must then question the general opinion we hold on sex, which on a chemical level is near-identical. To quote Hill, our nature towards sex is of "open season" as we further distance ourselves from the importance of moderation and focus on moderating other stimuli. This showcases a societal hypocrisy, a clear contradiction on a stimulus which is pushed aside and hidden because we only recently were liberated in the matter. So to acknowledge danger would appear on the surface as reversing progress.

This liberation didn't expect a coincidental rise of the internet (pornography) and hence the quagmire of a situation. Previously, in "The Stoic Palate", we spoke about satiation, the concept of pleasure versus satisfaction; satisfaction being the consumption of food and the pleasure being experienced through "the chase". I think that more people are realising that with sexual pleasure the "pleasure period" requires no resources and so the satisfaction can come within very short periods of time, making it one more dangerous for attachment but with less proof externally (as there's no complementary belly to show).

It could be that we are focused too much on aestheticism in the modern world, which allows sexual dependency to slip by. The previous strict sexual mores of Christianity are no longer part of popular culture, so to restrict sexuality seems like we are moving backwards. Yet this freedom has potential for abuse. The more closely aligned an act is to the survival of our lives the more difficult it is for us to accept the notion that it can be bad. Sex *is* important, but it's not as important as food, as we can survive day to day without it. Of course, sex is necessary for procreation – and orgasm is the most euphoric natural experience possible. Sex is verboten, almost taboo to many – not in the act itself, but in *revoking* the act. Restraint is difficult to embrace (more so for men) because the "achievement" of sex is socially rewarded.

Sexual pleasure is a desire that some claim is the essential purpose of life: procreation. So where do we draw the line and decide whether abstaining from any type of sexual pleasure is the most virtuous decision? The Epicureans hold an ambivalent attitude and the Stoics teach us to resist this urge on the basis of preserving reason. Diogenes Laërtius explains that: "Pleasure is an irrational elation over what seems to be worth choosing; under it are ranged enchantment, mean-spirited satisfaction, enjoyment, rapture. Enchantment is a pleasure which charms one through the sense of hearing; mean-spirited satisfaction is pleasure at someone else's misfortunes; enjoyment is, as it were, a turning, a kind of incitement of the soul to slackness; rapture is a breakdown of virtue."

When we indulge in a sexual urge and climax without the intent of procreating we are diminishing our ability to think and act rationally in the very act of submission to this desire. One could even argue that sexual activity for recreation is the very antithesis of living in accordance to nature and reason. Biologically, we are identical to our recent past, but clearly on a societal level the contemporary sexual paradigm has shifted.

So is it in our best interest to live in accordance to a belief that may seem outdated? To support this viewpoint one could consider the copious clinically backed facts about having regular sex, such as heart health, lowered blood pressure, increased libido, good form of exercise, increased intimacy and bonding, reduced risk of prostate cancer and even an improved immunity. So shouldn't we respect this as proof of sex being a good thing? Isn't intentional restriction therefore the most irrational option? Well, maybe.

Sex is something humans will do anyway. Restriction doesn't favour evolution-driven behaviour, this is clear. A healthy meal has many benefits: it is nourishing, full of nutrients, and in this adds value to one's life. However, with too many calories on a frequent basis (despite being "healthy food") this can lead to problems similar to those caused by a moderate intake of unhealthy food. This is the same with sex. Yes, perhaps it is unwise to align food and sex as absolute analogies to one another as there are other variables which must be taken into account (gender, love and bonding). However, what is clear is that there is an issue on the rise. According to the Society for the Advancement of Sexual Health, around 3–5 per cent of the US population (nine million) meet the requirements for sexual addiction.

The way I see Stoic love, it's being able to cherish those close to you, including your lover. The way you cherish your lover is doing so without the permeable wall in place between this love which allows for irrational passion to take place and disturb your tranquillity. Now you may decide that in order to experience greater *eudaimonia* you are going to abstain from sex completely because you believe this will increase your overall pleasure. It might, if the decision you are making diametrically opposes what you have done for a prolonged period of time. For instance, you might think that that having sex will decrease your pleasure because afterwards you will crave it. Or you might temporarily give up such things as a Stoic exercise so that you don't fear the uncertainty of a future lack of them. These make sense, but should not equate to a "thou shall not" and should be more applicable to the situation you find yourself in right now.

The real question is, are you acting *justly* in the sexual act? For instance, is it causing mental or emotional (or even physical) harm to someone else? No good. Is it completely mutual with "no strings attached"? That's okay. Or are you lusting after someone you shouldn't? Seneca warns us that pursuing pleasures "is like pursuing a wild beast: on being captured, it can turn on us and tear us to pieces". Epictetus clarifies that our dominating desire is to cease desiring what we know we cannot actually accomplish.

It would appear that "not all orgasms are made the same". Wide empirical evidence has made it clear that the benefits listed above for sex are not the same for masturbation. Furthermore, it is easier to become dependent and attached to this act for the simple fact that investment and willingness to overcome discomfort is not needed. ("Investment and willingness" implies courtship and effort). This effort is fulfilled through a medium (such as pornography) which acts as an "evolutionary hack", a shortcut, if you will. Although a slightly distasteful example, sex versus masturbation is analogous to cooking your own meal versus buying fast food.

I once heard some say: "A guy who doesn't work out, is lazy, does nothing worthwhile and lives life as an unjust man has the ability to trick his brain into thinking he is getting more sex, love and affection than the most powerful clan leader alive thousands of years ago – all with the click of a button." Again, not politically correct, but this represents the disconnect and dissonance in the natural flow of events which precede genuine human relationships. Pornography has provided, on a global scale, a paradigm of ease of access to a progression in life which naturally requires discomfort and effort.

We admit sex is desirable! But at the end of the day, this all comes down to self-sufficiency. Ask yourself: at what point is this pleasurable act in your life causing you to be dependent, for it is the dependency to pleasure which dissolves tranquillity, *not the pleasure itself.*

PART EIGHT:
THE BIGGER PICTURE

"I tell you, because military training is not publicly recognised by the state, you must not make that an excuse for being a whit less careful in attending to it yourself. For you may rest assured that there is no kind of struggle, apart from war, and no undertaking in which you will be worse off by keeping your body in better fettle."

– Socrates

THE DAWN OF CIVILISATION

Pre-10,000 BC primate nomadic lifestyles were based around hunting and gathering. One of the most dramatic shifts in the evolution of humanity was the Neolithic Agricultural Revolution which occurred around 10,000-8000 BC. During the dawn of civilisation there was a switch in human behaviour from hunting and gathering to agriculture, settlement and the formation of large scale permanent establishments. Agriculture brought not only a revolution in how we sustain ourselves but also modification to the environment through crops, irrigation and deforestation. As we all know today, this advancement has come back to bite us.

In ancient China there was a philosophy which emphasised correctness of relationships, a high regard for justice and sincerity. This philosophy was called Confucius. Confucius was actually a traditional deity of Taoism, which some scholars see as the other side of the same coin as Stoicism. The teachings of Confucius encouraged followers to exercise on a regular basis. In the age of Confucius, the sedentary lifestyle was becoming more and more apparent. A disregard for physical movement was known as "organ malfunction" – perhaps we can equate this to cardiovascular disease. It became clear to humans at this time that exercise was important and this was shown through the Chinese people's wide variety of physical aptitudes including wrestling, archery and dance.

In this over-simplified history lesson, next came the Greeks (2500-200 BC). As we covered previously, Greeks idealised physical perfection as one of the epitomes of their culture. As the founders of the Olympics, no other society held the prowess of physical excellence in such high regard. Music was also important. "Exercise for the body and music for the soul" was a common phrase. Training for young boys occurred in the *palaestra*, later in the gymnasium – typically between the ages of fourteen and sixteen –where they were supervised by a *paidotribe* (the equivalent to a personal trainer).

The rise of the Roman Empire came through mass conquest between the third century BC and the third century AD. Looking back into the earlier days of Rome, around 400 BC, it's perplexing to think about how these people carved out one of the greatest empires of all time. What was interesting about Roman civilisation was that physical training peaked during times of conflict and the expansion of the empire. Since all men between the ages of seventeen and sixty were eligible for conscription into the military they would have to remain in peak condition to secure the welfare of themselves and others. The result? A civilisation that went on to conquer most of the Western world.

Romulus Augustalus (born AD 460 and died some time after 527 AD) was the last of the Roman emperors in the west and was easily overthrown by the Germanic leader Flavius Odoacer (AD 433–493) who became the first barbarian to rule over Rome. The complex ideas surrounding the true reasons behind the collapse of Rome are still debated and discussed today as these ideas are still relevant to the modern discourse surrounding state failure.

Stoicism was very influential on Christianity, and contributed to the thought of many other philosophical figures in the following centuries – particularly Baruch Spinoza, Thomas More and René Descartes. Although these modern figures were influenced greatly by Stoicism there were certainly cases where they opposed one another. Baruch Spinoza (1632-1677) held much of the same beliefs as the Stoics in regards to happiness, but where he differed sharply was that he rejected the notion that rationale can defeat emotion. In more recent times we have come to see the likes of Cognitive Behavioural Therapy (CBT) which has its foundation in Stoicism. I highly recommend Donald Robertson's *The Philosophy of Cognitive Behavioural Therapy*.

Stoicism itself was popularised and born in a world which essentially was falling apart. After the death of Alexander the Great, the philosophy of Stoicism offered the people security in a time of hardship. With the fall of the Roman Empire came the rise of Christianity and while Stoicism itself was a philosophy which persisted through time and influenced the education of Roman aristocracy, according to Gilbert Murray, who wrote *The Stoic Philosophy* in 1915, there's no evidence to suggest that the philosophy was still part of Rome's political culture or to the transitory emperors which later would come to power.

In AD 529 Emperor Justinian (AD 482 – 565) shut down

the philosophical schools, and subsequently philosophy become more of a subject of academia, as the schools contradicted the society Emperor Justinian envisioned. The moral merits of the philosophy, although praised in some sense, were attributed to the influence from the Christian deity. According to Massimo Pigliucci, there are several explanations for the decline. Pigliucci outlines the fact that Roman society had simply changed too much. And there was a lack of teachers with the charisma of Musonius or Epictetus. With the success of the Roman Empire came a decline into comfort as victors, especially in the latter part of the Roman Empire. The emperors and their underlings entertained themselves with material acquisition and hedonistic behaviours. They believed that they ruled the world – which may have been true – but their flaw was that they denied any danger of retribution from external forces. Clearly they were wrong, and when Barbarian Flavius Odoacer took charge, it was too late.

Like the Romans, we have relaxed into the same path they followed. If history is correct in predicting the future then I say we are experiencing the same weakness and vulnerability that the Romans did. Not necessarily to the invasion of another emperor, but perhaps an even more dangerous foe: ourselves.

THE CIVILIAN

It's clear that there has been a dramatic decline since 1999 of sugar/refined carbohydrate intake per person in the US, but also much of the Western world. This data comes from the *National Health and Nutrition Examination* surveys. Despite sugar clearly being an innate driver for survival, and part of most people's poor dietary decisions, there must be other variables influencing the exponential growth of obesity. Is it inherently fattening? No. Is it a large contributing factors to obesity and diet driven disease? Yes. More than 38 per cent of the United States population is categorised as obese, and the majority of the Western world mirrors this trend. But what is the deeper cause of overeating?

What first comes to mind is our sedentary lifestyle. This is self-explanatory. Sugar is decreasing while obesity is increasing; so therefore our increased technological development and lifestyle must be compensating for the gap. You may argue that it's the rise of high fructose corn syrup which is the problem. But once again, contrary to common belief, there's a lack of evidence for HFCS being the cause of obesity, according to a 2013 review from the *International Journal of Obesity*. The use of HFCS rapidly increased from 1970 to 1999, mostly as a replacement for sucrose. Its use peaked around 1999 and has been falling since.

There's something else, something pervasive and persistent in our culture's philosophy – something deeper than sugar. Although never to be completely excluded as a contributing factor, we must think on a deeper level. Perhaps we should consider *why* we manufacture something like artificial sweeteners in the first place and the mindset which led to this being the "rational" course of action.

There isn't much we can do to make people exercise more, other than hammer the importance of physical movement through education, and by using different methods (an example being physical video games). The point is that many are unaware just how dangerous sedentary habits are and most lack the awareness to understand how significant the change has been through the last decade. But once again I think we *must* look deeper; there *must* be a deeper reason which has provoked the age of the coach potato.

With such a complex issue it seems too vague to exclude any other variables from having any worthwhile impact on this trend. I argue much like the shift from war, strength and military might to materialistic, hedonism and relaxed celebration is occurring right now. We are lacking a reason to live that extends beyond the self. If you're reading this you're likely a civilian. Perhaps you are or were in the military, but chances are you are a civilian. You are part of a standard urban society and you work, study and are well-immersed in the liberal, democratic and free culture of the Western world. But just *how* thankful should we be to have so much dominion over our own lifestyle? The body of a man whose call to war is out of his control must not only be ready for his own well-being, as this desire is selfish. For soldiers the strength and capacity of your body to endure pain and discomfort is also for the selfless care of fellow comrades in warfare. The lack of discipline of one man may very well lead to the death of another. Reliance is key and teamwork fundamental for victory and survival. For the standard civilian, this attitude is not upheld in daily life.

If we examine the animal kingdom, it is clear that all organisms are proficient in self-preservation, and are designed to fulfil their own needs. According to the Stoics, as we age we become more selfless, and value giving to the world and to our wider circle. This was known as *oikeiôsis*, meaning our self-ownership. The idea is that at a certain age humans will utilise reason as a means to dominate over their impulse as the governor of self-management. After the years of complete self-interest as a child, we extend ourselves for our families, communities, countries and the entire universe itself. As I mentioned previously in the introduction, the Stoics emphasised this sort of ethical obligation to serve our wider community.

Do we give people the opportunity to fulfil this altruistic desire to serve one's country which was previously fulfilled through war? If we specifically look at Western countries and other highly developed regions of the world with an obesity problem (the United States, New Zealand, Australia, Canada, the United Kingdom), we see these countries have one variable in common – no mandatory military conscription. Now, correlation doesn't equal causation, and the point isn't to reach a consensus on the significance of this correlation (this is up to further research), but if history is correct then there's at least some truth to this idea.

An example of a factor that could give us the impression that military service is not directly attributed to the increase in obesity prevalence is that the nations which require military service are less developed, less wealthy and citizens don't have the freedom to make the *privileged* decision to overeat when sustenance is merely a form of survival.

Singapore is a fascinating example of a country, industrialised and first tier, with low levels of obesity. Post-basic training Singaporean men are required to devote some time every year to stay fit and able for the IPPT (Individual Physical Proficiency Test), which tests all men on the basic components of motor and physical condition. These tests include standing broad jumps, chin-ups and a 2.4 km run.

Worldwide, the prevalence of the overweight and the obese varies significantly. Overall, more women are obese than men. The disparity of the obese favouring women is especially pronounced in developing regions of the world, namely, Africa and the Middle East. According to the Centers for Disease Control, in the developed world more men are overweight – and thus at risk for obesity – than women. In the ten years from 1999, obesity increased rapidly in men but not women. In 1999, in the United States, 27.5 per cent of men were obese, while 33.4 per cent of women were obese. In 2009, 35.8 per cent of women were obese, only a slight increase of 2.4 per cent. For men, however, the rate of obesity had shot up to 35.5 per cent by 2009 – an increase of 8 per cent, and a difference of 5.6 per cent between the genders. These figures are alarming, not only because of the population size involves; but also because such a change happened even while males have a greater propensity for leaner physiques due to their hormonal profile. The reason why we see such a disproportion for more obese women in the developing world is speculated to be because of fat being a sign of fertility to many cultures and ironically a sign of healthfulness and prosperity (which it is to an extent) but clearly a dangerous dogma to hold as an absolute.

Perhaps this is a reflection of the absence of the need to

serve and protect, and the feminisation of healthy. A "desire to serve their country" implies a country is at war, which most Western countries are not. Contrary to common belief, wide empirical evidence suggests we live in the most peaceful era ever when we look at worldwide battle deaths per 100,000 people. We just presume it is violent, as social media shows us that bad stuff the moment we roll out of bed.

Stoics were certainly not pacifists. For the Stoic, the refusal or acceptance of serving in battle was subjective to whether one option served humanity or not. Stoic writers wrote about killing, and sometimes what was conducive to their philosophy involved war. Seneca, in *On Anger*, believes that he is ordering the death of men; but he does it with the correct attitude. The founder of Stoicism, Zeno, apparently died by suffocating himself after falling and breaking his toe. From the beginning, suicide and violence were not foreign concepts to the classical Stoics.

The Art of War is an incredibly informative book on war and strategy written by Sun Tzu, a Chinese general. The underlying moral of his book is war itself is a bad omen and peace is the ideal solution – very similar to the position of the Stoics.

Anyway, back to the point. We mostly live in safety and so it raises the question: do we actually need to be fit for any reason other than living a healthier life? You can argue that you cannot force someone to *want* to be healthy and fit in the long term, despite the enforcement of physical duty. I would argue that enforcing discipline would allow some to see the benefit of self-control and therefore increase the likelihood of them adhering to such a mindset. What is clear is that when this need is lost people can get too comfortable, and life begins to revolve around seeking out pleasure. To be candid, you don't have to be able to squat a certain percentage of your body weight, or adhere to three gym training sessions per week, in order to be able to perform data entry in an office. Any fatigue brought on by an unhealthy lifestyle can be mitigated through drugs, or so it would seem – so what's the point? Why ignore temptation and practise self-control when you're still going to be living a "reasonable life", even if it is hedonistic by nature?

What is the solution then? Mass conscription to the military and propaganda to instigate violent conflict abroad to create a sense of urgency so "Max" can get ready for the beach? Of course not.

Negative Visualisation

The Stoics called negative visualisation "the premeditation of evils". Modern clinical psychologists may refer to it as *defensive pessimism*. Psychologist Julie Norem says defensive pessimism is a strategy used regularly by between 25–30 per cent of Americans. Author and entrepreneur Tim Ferris truly popularised this in the modern world of business, reconstructing the idea of negative visualisation and labelling it *practical pessimism*. Recent studies have now recognised the merits of using negative moods strategically, as seen in the 2013 study from *Sage Journals* (a fitting name) called, "Don't Worry, Be Sad!" In this study, psychologists confirmed that mild bad moods – which are often unconscious – promote an attentive and detailed style of thinking, which is useful in difficult situations.

To better understand how intentional negative visualisations can work to help create a sense of urgency, let's take a look at some of the richest, most privileged people in the world; the classical example being celebrities. These people live up to society's aspirations in the image of "success." We can then approach the question of why do many of these people who have the life we have always dreamed of constantly drown their sorrows in the same short-term gratifying habits aligned to the lowest parts of society.

We can compare this to the freedom of your discipline and temperance. The choice simply becomes choosing a path of progression or degeneration; moving forwards or backwards. The freedom is there; the choice is yours and this freedom of choice becomes the catalyst for potential regression. In today's world, this practical pessimism becomes more important than ever, and we must reaffirm hypothetical scenarios which reinforce our urgency to do justice to ourselves.

Negative visualisation is the meditative exercise of intentionally bringing the worst contemplations to the self. The Stoic would focus and meditate on the loss of loved ones, assets, even their own limbs, in an effort to create a state of appreciation and gratitude. Going back to military conscription and war, we can compare this state of mind to the underlying urgency and motive a solider has towards his ability to train the body in order to improve his chances of survival, as well as the survival of his comrades and country.

The hedonic cycle provides a clear representation for most people's belief systems today.

- We strive to accomplish our desires.
- When achieved, we quickly lose satisfaction.
- This fuels a greater desire for more.

It is damaging to always ponder on what we don't have and what we want. Contrary to the media-fuelled positivity revolution we can make healthier choices through a direct appreciation and examination of what we don't have through this practical pessimism. You can do so in your premeditations and evening retrospections going through scenarios similar to those below:

- If you don't want to eat a healthy meal? Visualise your life as a constant struggle to steal food as your money is all going to your family's survival.
- If you don't want to train your legs? Visualise your legs broken and your body handicapped, prisoned in a wheelchair forever.
- If you don't want to wake up early? Visualise your mornings as a time where you would live the life of a slave.

- If you stop halfway through barefoot running because it hurts? Visualise your fellow soldier dying at the hands of your perception of the pain.

Before a sprinting session or a gym session we can consider every possibility of the activity going wrong. For instance, before you do sprinting intervals you can contemplate on your calf muscle being pulled, or knee pain occurring after the training session. If we consider every possible situation, especially the *worst* possible, we are allowing ourselves to lower our expectations and thus not be as affected by these outcomes if they occur.

EUSTRESS VERSUS DISTRESS

Today it's very clear to us that our thoughts can embody significant chemical change in the body. If you think about something that provokes worry and uncertainty your stress is going to increase.

Cortisol (which you should now be familiar with) and adrenaline are stress hormones, and both are secreted in the adrenal glands. However, they function in different ways. While cortisol binds to fat cells, your pancreas and liver, adrenaline has a more direct effect on the contraction of your muscles and your heart rate (which increases with more adrenaline), also your respiration. From both a physiological and physiological perspective, increased adrenaline in the body will allow you to withstand more stressful activities as it is triggered by the sympathetic nervous system. Adrenaline is more commonly known through the overdramatic, cinematic scenes of injecting someone's jugular with adrenaline in order to save their life.

A 1998 study from the journal *Pain* looked at twenty-four people, twelve male and twelve female, to see whether adrenaline actually amplified pain. The results showed that adrenaline allows you to withstand stressful situation, but it isn't the variable which masks pain, as it is often said to be. The reduction of the perception of pain from negatively visualising your fellow soldier dying at your hands, or withstanding cold temperatures, is not due to adrenaline masking pain. It comes from the fact that your attention is diverted so strongly to other activities that the pain becomes irrelevant to you. Therefore, if you focus on pain, even with high levels of adrenaline you will still feel the pain and perhaps it will be pronounced. The fact that this is possible reaffirms what Marcus Aurelius once said about being distressed about those things which are external and how we have the power to revoke stress at any moment.

Negative visualisation may seem to contradict the previous section where I explained that we must decrease our cortisol levels and overall stress; but the practice of negative visualisation will benefit us in short bursts, as it is made up for by its long-lasting effects on our peace of mind. I would categorise this type of stress as being *eustress*, which, as I've mentioned before, means beneficial or "good" stress. This term was coined by endocrinologist Hans Selye, who explains that the difference between the "bad" (distress) and the "good" (eustress) is that distress leads to anxiety, withdrawals and states of sadness, while eustress can enhance an individual's function, despite both being equally taxing.

Some examples of eustress are the Wim Hof breathing method which is becoming increasingly popular, riding a roller coaster, exercise and of course, fasting/ketogenic diets and negative visualisation.

Similar to a soldier who has an innate sense of urgency, we can create our own urgency by being grateful through meditating on the negative areas of our psyche.

PRIVILEGE, WEALTH AND GRATITUDE

Stoicism becomes more important than ever as what is "privileged" and "rich" for our biological selves becomes abundant and expected. In a materialistic sense not everyone is rich, but to our genetic desires we are all wealthy. Taking into consideration fasting and "rehearsing poverty", it becomes obvious that those most in need of this practice for moral good are those who spend their lives validating their standard of success through wealth and other materialistic goods, when on a physiological sense they were rich all along. Stoicism becomes an important tool to humble those blind to the tranquillity freely available to them.

If we take the story of most blind people, they come to appreciate their "flaw" as something more closely resembling a gift. Some (but not all) who go blind find they become more aware of their other senses. In the event that something similar to this would occur to you (such as conscription into war and likely death) you would be more ready to deal with the reality of it. If you can genuinely formulate these visualisations and are convincing and persuasive to yourself, virtue through tranquillity of the mind is the inevitable consequence. Negative visualisation is *not* to promote an anxious and depressive state. There is a difference between exploring the negative and attaching yourself to the possibility through fear and worry.

THE DISCOMFORT OF UNCERTAINTY

> "There are only a few who control themselves
> and their affairs by a guiding purpose; the rest
> do not proceed; they are merely swept along,
> like objects afloat in a river."
>
> – Seneca

DETERMINISM AND FATE

Our firstly priority should be examination of ourselves. Seneca tells us business is next; then comes those who are affected by our acts (don't mistake this for selfishness). Care for ourselves is selfless as this leads to care for others. We ought to have an adequate and accurate (as far as possible) estimation of ourselves, our potential and capabilities, as too often we can fail through our arrogance. Some demand more from their mind and others through tasks that wear down a weakening body. There is greater strength in the bearer than in the burden of an act itself.

The archer is a key Stoic analogy which gives us the opportunity to explore how we can define what we call "goals" today. The archer's mastery of the bow and arrow represents the flaw with the contemporary definition of a goal. This flaw is why people fail to realise their ambitions. This isn't to say that Stoicism itself isn't a compatible philosophy with the ambitious and goal oriented, rather that we must understand how fate interacts with our ambitions and wishes. Every archer will draw his bow to the best of his ability and let it go with the most calculated and accurate release possible. The trust in repeated practice and skill of the archer is everything in this moment, but it doesn't entirely define the success or whether the target is hit. After the arrow is released, its course is determined no longer by the skill of the archer, but by the nature of the external world. The harsh winds and other extremes all control the direction of the arrow and the likelihood it will pierce its target. A gust of the wind is out of control of the archer; no matter how skilled he may be, the arrow will *always* be vulnerable to the fatalism of nature. Hitting the target is preferred but not desired.

You may ask, if everything is reliant on fate, then why do anything? This is a common argument against fate, called "the lazy argument". Chrysuppus' reply was that everything is co-fated. For example, type 2 diabetes is provoked prematurely by unhealthy choices you make. The Stoics were compatibilists. This means that to the Stoics, fate and free will don't conflict with one another.

Innately we love goals. They provide us with satisfaction among the uncertainty of life. Contrary to our fondness in setting them, and our optimism in the moment of writing them down, the follow-through can often bring dissatisfaction and feelings of inadequacy. Often this experience of inadequacy is followed by a deepening of the void. Despite constant setbacks and failures to attain our goals, we still continue to set them due to this overbearing uncertainty. Often at times we become too arrogant in what we can realistically achieve. I would say this occurs in moments of more extreme melancholy where uncertainty is more pronounced than ever.

With every long-term or short-term goal, you must stop and think about what is going to precede this action, and most importantly, what the consequence will be. In the *Enchiridion*, Epictetus speaks about a scenario where a man wishes to win at Olympia, further explaining how great an accomplishment this would indeed be. What a man must do before submitting to the *discipline* and *work* such a goal would require is to consider the first movements he will make. A man should contemplate the reality that he will not touch any sweets; training when he wishes to rest will be routine; and his free will is handed to the man who will train him. With this submission comes the very real risk of hurting himself, twisting his arm, dislocating him shoulder, and all the while still losing the competition! It is only after one has truly and honestly considered these variables that a goal should be sought after.

With this contemplation comes your commitment to take action towards the act and with such commitment comes your best efforts. By contrast, the man who acts out of emotion will find the pursuit will lead to nothing but a half-hearted attempt – as it is merely one of many undertakings.

As you know by now, some things are clearly in our control and others not. Those in our control are our opinions, our desires, our aversions. Out of control are our bodies, reputation and the material world. Metaphysically, Stoics are determinists in the sense that there are no consequences or changes which aren't dictated by a chain of events or specific causes. The Stoics do have a concept which one may call chance, but this was more in reference to a measure of human ignorance. "Random" events are those which happen beyond the comprehension of human beings.

In Stoic physics there is a distinction made between "principle" and "antecedent" causes (antecedent simply being the cause which logically precedes another). If we take cause 1, cause 2, cause 3 and cause 4, then cause 1 is the antecedent of 3 and 2 being the principle.

Providence is often described as God's intervention in the world. This idea is widely debated among various modern Stoic scholars, often cited as the so-called debate of "providence or atoms". For some, this is a central question to life. My opinion, for what it's worth, is simply that I feel that, overall, it doesn't matter – in the context of *The Stoic Body* – Stoicism works regardless. To put it bluntly, who gives a damn? It's the practicality of the philosophy and living life for that matter which should be prioritised and emphasised. As I previously mentioned, the Stoics preferred to *do* over *think*. As Pierre Hadot writes, "Either providence – in which case we must live like Stoics – or else atoms – in which case we still have to live like Stoics."

The wise Stoic is able to tackle whatever the world throws at him regardless because, as Stoics understand it, how the universe works as a rational system, and who governs this system, is irrelevant to the pragmatic and practical nature valued by Stoics. What the Stoics certainly did *not* believe in is the Christian-like mysterious workings of God's plan, only achievable through salvation.

The Stoics do believe in God, but that the universe itself is God. Chrysippus affirms that "the universe itself is God and the universal outpouring of its soul." Scholars often describe the "religion" of the Stoics as a form of *pantheism*. Famous Pantheists include Albert Einstein and Alan Watts. Chrysippus clarified his beliefs by explaining that gods make up different aspects of an entire universe. Cicero told us that "he further maintained that aether is that which people call Zeus, and that the air which permeates the seas is Poseidon, and that the earth is what is known by the name of Demeter, and he treated in similar style the names of the other gods."

This planetary body we call earth is a place which is built for its owners, not humanity which inhabits it. Fate, destiny, providence, fatalism, Zeus's will – whatever you want to call it – these terms describe the reality that everything is essentially subject to contingency. The Stoics had a great mechanism for dealing with this, because some may develop the attitude of "what's the point" or "why should I care about my health or being fit". It's easy to slip into the mindset of the ambivalent, the nihilistic and hold nothing but embitterment towards a world which at times does not respond to your hopes.

GOALS WORTHY OF A PHILOSOPHER

Before I cover exactly what an appropriate goal for a Stoic looks like, we must understand that Stoicism is firstly priori-tised on setting goals worthy of a philosopher. The wisdom from the past is not necessarily going to give us a specific "how-to formula" on the best step-by-step method to set goals. This is especially true if goals orientate around the superfluous (as many people's goals are). First and foremost our goals are to be better people; then health, as this *may* help us to become greater people; to then act as better people. This is the reason why I believe Seneca and Marcus Aurelius felt so compelled to become a part of Roman government, and also why Epictetus and Musonius felt such a compelling desire to teach the doctrine of Stoicism. They intended to make it clear that despite the complementary nature of goals and a Stoic mindset, the philosophy itself is far from being founded upon *aiming* for massive achievement; this would be a contradiction to your priorities. As cliché as it sounds, the *journey* is what is important. The successes which come after are the by-product of virtue being upheld on a consistent basis.

The individual decisions we make in the present are what

define whether a goal is to be labelled as one worthy of a philosopher. Goals are sought after through methodical and systematic approaches in order to fulfil a specific objective. Essentially all we can do is apply the "reserve clause" to take its course as we reason and rationalise our decisions one at a time.

To put this idea into a practical scenario: imagine you have a goal of deadlifting 180 kg in 12 weeks' time (increasing it from your current maximum of 140 kg). Let's say you increase your strength but fail to achieve the objective number of 180 kg and only reach 170 kg. To define exactly what a goal is we must ask the question: "Have I failed to achieve the goal?" With the contemporary understanding of the word goal, the answer is, "Of course I did." You did not meet the objective aim (you did not reach the 180 kg) so you *failed* to achieve the goal.

But is this the ideal approach for a wise man? I say this is in fact the worst possible mindset you can have. If you only reached 170 kg, but through the "journey" and the process of accumulating strength through your disciplines you lived in virtue and made just decisions, then surely punishing yourself for being unable to reach an arbitrary number reinforces the normalcy of living for exercise instead of exercising to live. Many people will obsessively write to-do lists to cultivate certainty for every step of their day. This can give your life an almost robot-like experience and the more we plan and fill this discomfort through our expectations of what we wish to happen, we are simply antagonising a force of fate which is undoubtedly going to be the victor.

"The Sage does not change his decision, if everything remains entirely what it was when he took it …. Elsewhere, however, he undertakes everything "with a reserve clause" … in his most steadfast decisions, he allows for uncertain events."

– Seneca

A skilled gardener will trim flowers from the bush in order to allow the bigger and stronger flowers to blossom and bloom. Be the gardener of your life and make the reasoned decision to choose the right "flowers" to grow. Which sprouts from your plant are holding back the potential growth of others? Ignore how alluring their beauty and fragrance may be. Likewise, the best travel experiences are usually those of spontaneity. When someone plans their itinerary but things change, you have to adapt and do something different. The goal isn't specifically in the objective pursuit but in the knowledge that you are free to travel.

Powerful goals come from recognising that we are strong and directional like the release of an arrow but we are also vulnerable to the forces of wind. Do not oppose nature as nothing good will come from this act. Fire your arrow with direction, authority and conviction – but don't be so arrogant as to deny the very real probability that nature's wind will challenge the course of your preconceived hope. Hope itself represents a sort of emotive investment in future circumstances. By itself it's not enough to simply have hope if you have aims to achieve, but we must also be happy despite the outcome.

Marcus Aurelius gives us the example of bread; he explains that even the small things produced by nature are attractive and pleasing in their own way. Bread rises as it cooks, then some cracks, splits and openings appear on the surface of the bread. These parts which break open do so in accordance to nature and often it is contrary to the art and intention of the baker, but the wise baker is still happy to eat the bread. I argue the wisest baker holds an even greater appreciation for the peculiar nature of the broken bread – as what charm is there with predictability? Be secure in the person you're becoming, instead of the outcome.

Nomos

The Stoics were especially interested in adopting rules, rather than objective "goals" for living a virtuous life. The fascinating thing about rules is that they make life simple, while goals can complicate your life but appear simple on the surface. The best way to approach "rules" is to strictly live by them and obey what you have set for yourself. Through setting well thought out rules and following them, you are essentially cultivating a path which is more likely to fortify virtuous acts despite how the metaphorical wind may disturb your arrow. Examples of rules could be: thirty minutes of reading per day, morning premeditations, evening retrospections, going to every gym session possible (without a valid excuse), or a minimum of 7.5 hours of sleep.

Now, these can be called "goals" in themselves, but goal itself implies there's an end. These rules fit under the goal of "being healthier" or "getting fitter" which by themselves are extremely vague and imply less possibility of action ever being taken on a consistent basis. In the *Enchiridion*, Epictetus tells us that for whatever moral rules we place for ourselves, they are to be obeyed as if they were laws. Therefore, your moral rules should be carefully selected and changed only if truly necessary. When you have rules to live by, it makes decision-making simple for the small things, which allows the mind to ponder on topics of greater importance. So set these laws as if your life is the world and your dominion is the government. Legislation is not decided overnight.

Always consider the implications of enforcing or revoking laws in your life. As mundane as they seem, again, to paraphrase Zeno, these rules or little things are nevertheless no little thing in themselves. Your rules don't all need to be and implemented at the same time. Adopt one major rule at a time. There are some rules which will require a change in your environment, while others will focus more on needing accountability.

One should never live a life revolved around athletics. Even though Seneca and various other Stoic philosophers clearly valued the use of physical exercise and healthy food, their reasoning behind this differs from today's health and fitness industry and likewise you too have the dominion to make your own choice, but for what it's worth, Seneca's view on this articulates the underlying narrative of *The Stoic Body*. It's not that Stoic doctrine rejects physical exercise, far from it. But Seneca always remained perplexed at the fact that so many men were willing to sacrifice the comfort of their body, through agonising, even obsessive training; but so few spent nearly enough time putting their mind and spiritual nature through the same aggression, pain and suffering.

If you willingly sacrifice your life in the pursuit of athletic feats, your days will revolve around these physical challenges when the act is based on nothing of value. I remember a friend of mine who, after years of never exercising or caring about his health, joined the gym, ate healthier and was on top of the world. It gave him drive and a purpose for living, similar to the "honeymoon" phase of a relationship. With time, this ended and old habits resurfaced; testimony to why you should never allow your focus to be solely on the body.

DOING OVER THINKING

I think as we progress we must appreciate different "styles" of being Stoic. The purists must hate the idea. I say we separate and make a distinction between the old and the new. This is not to degrade classical Stoicism, but to do what makes sense and adapt for modern times. As Stoic expert Professor Christopher Gill points out, Epictetus was a strict man, leaning towards the Cynic model of quasi-asceticism. Musonius, as I have mentioned, was seen as a progressive but also a conservative man. I covered this idea of "styles" of Stoicism earlier in this book in my discussion on deontology and how Stoicism will never be such a philosophy. One could be vegan, one could be omnivorous; but neither determine whether one is considered a Stoic.

A point I'd like to finish on is on Stoics being "doers" rather than "ponderers". It was Epictetus who had a disdain for the theoretical philosophy as we find in the *Discourses*. He said: "We know how to analyse arguments, and have the skill a person needs to evaluate competent logicians. But in life what do I do? What today I say is good, tomorrow I will swear is bad. And the reason is that, compared to what I know about syllogisms, my knowledge and experience of life fall far behind".

Once you understand what *virtue* means, once you understand what to do, then do it. Don't theorise; read to the extent where you dismiss time where you could be actively living as the Stoic himself and receiving the reward for what you contemplate receiving. When you keep arguing back and forth and the argument becomes so esoteric then you get comfortable in the push-pull of the discourse and lose grasp of your willpower. This is perhaps similar to the constant arguments in nutrition and exercise occurring in spite of time itself.

A great quote I was told at one point went something like this: "Reading books is great, but there has to be a point in a man's life where he stops reading and starts writing." In this case, writing is not the point; writing is analogous to *actually* doing, taking action and putting theory into practice. Consider Marcus Aurelius' admonition: "No longer talk at all about the kind of man that a good man ought to be, but be such."

It is fascinating to recognise that the Stoics' naturalistic account of moral behaviours and virtue expressed through (fasting, voluntary discomforts, negative visualisations, remaining detached, etc) are parallel in agreement to modern cognitive research and what is being rediscovered. It's tempting to make assumptions about their deeper technical knowledge, but this would be an anachronistic interpretation and least we forget most original accounts of Stoic thought are lost forever. We live in a strange world where we become so technical and detail oriented in the pursuit of finding a deeper meaning in nature when the answer is right in front of us. Live consistently and in accordance with nature and the answers you need will reveal themselves to you.

EPILOGUE
MEMENTO MORI

Death doesn't make life pointless, death makes life worth living. The world keeps spinning when you're gone. So many of us live life with an attitude which represents the arrogant thought that we are destined to live forever. Your life is in an hour glass and the hole which that sand is pouring through could widen or break at any moment.

Death is natural and inevitable. What happens after death is up for discussion; but the fact remains that nobody can trick or bypass this inevitability. Our very discomfort and fear with the concept of death leads people to follow a morally bad path. If you're young or old, male or female; whatever your age or wealth, status, position in life, your health should be of value to you. It is not valuable enough to sacrifice virtue for, but is valuable enough to do *something* about it.

Recently I was in Greece visiting family. After a short visit to Athens I made my way south-west on a bus to Argos, the home town of my mother's family. We went to visit my great-uncle, who was now in his mid to late eighties. The first thing we asked him was, "How are you?" and he replied, "Waiting…" It was clear he was waiting for death.

Life is short; we all know that. We're all aware that this isn't forever. Allow this truth to bring forth an inner joy for life and an urgency to *live* it. This starts with your virtue, and in my opinion health, discipline and temperance is a great path for many.

Stoicism is an ever-changing philosophy.

If we revert back to Epictetus and his Dichotomy of Control, the idea is basically that there's a strict (many argue almost too strict) division between what is and what isn't under our control. Preferred indifference (health, wealth, fame) relate to something we should strive to obtain, but never elevate to a virtue as they are external. Health can help us be in a more suitable environment for virtue to take place. But of course we are always prey to ailments and disease which are fundamentally outside of our control. I think that *The Stoic Body* calls for a new category, one where we elevate health to an "extremely preferred indifferent", prioritised over wealth and fame. Now of course having more fame usually means more money and more money *can* mean greater potential for health – and also the opposite. Likewise health can also become bad, as I covered with the Adonis Complex. But because lack of good health in today's age is disproportionate, by far, I think it seems reasonable to appreciate the value of health slightly more over wealth and fame (but of course it is not, nor will it ever be a virtue).

One night, when I was on a late night walk to the convenience store to buy a sandwich, I was inspired by something I heard. I entered the store and went to look at the selection of sandwiches. What I noticed was that two of them were priced cheaper. I grabbed the bacon and egg sandwich and as I approached the store clerk to pay for the food he told me that it's probably not a good idea to buy it. Naturally I questioned his response and he went on to say that they were expired by three days.

He said, "I have this friend back home. He is worth $2 million, he's young, has a beautiful wife and a successful business, but his health is bad and he can't enjoy any of it.

Pick another sandwich and for an extra dollar you may prevent illness for a few days."

This story very much reminded me of Marcus Aurelius' reference to cucumbers where he said: "Is your cucumber bitter? Throw it away. Are there briars in your path? Turn aside. That is enough. Do not go on and say, 'Why were things of this sort ever brought into this world?'"

We question why such things exist in the world. Instead we should just make the decision to throw the sandwich away, or turn away from the briars. This is enough. To ponder on the *why* will do nothing but have you ridiculed in the presence of a wise man. To think for even one moment why the sandwich had expired, or the cucumber was bitter is, in my eyes, disrespecting how you value your time. Thinking back, it's just a sandwich, but the underlying message behind the store clerk's advice is relevant, not only for the importance of health but for how much we can take our health for granted in a world which allows us to live off of our evolutionary autopilot. Always remember that no matter who you are, what your abilities are, or your "status", you can learn something valuable from *anybody*. This is one of the most important lessons I've ever learned.

To think about death and to fear it is irrational. You kill your ability to thrive; instead you simply cope. As Seneca said, "You are younger; but what does that matter? There is no fixed count of our years. You do not know where death awaits you; so be ready for it everywhere." As your eyes recognise the meaning of these words, as your mind absorbs the information from this page, as you breathe in and exhale, within the few seconds that have passed since you began this sentence, someone has likely died. They may have died from disease, old age or some unforeseen incident. Take a moment to think about how *you* perceive death in your life. Do you fear it? Now two more seconds have passed. Do you treasure *this very moment* and the air you breathe? These few seconds may very well be your last.

Our life should not be judged on the basis of its quantity; we must judge a man's life on his commitment to virtue. Today, gluttony, obesity and laziness are more abundant than ever as man's will to fight his desires and temptations dissipates. A groupthink mentality has created a world where our evolutionary desires are being fulfilled at an alarming rate. We live with heavy chains holding us back from living as we should. We are living a conflicting nature. Life is broken into stages. We are born, we die – and the stage in-between is what we call living. Separated into years, months, days, hours, minutes and seconds. The wise man chooses to focus attention on the seconds and regress into years. Most do the opposite.

I'm not the most muscular guy, I also don't lift the heaviest weights and I don't hold a world record. Chances are neither will you. But what I do have is confidence in my discipline, and that can never be taken away from me. You, too, will become confident in your discipline and self-control, which will last a lifetime if you follow the steps I have provided in *The Stoic Body*. What I also know is that this would have been so difficult for me to achieve without undergoing the discomforts and methods I wrote out in this book. From my years as a teenager gamer, playing computer games all day, without purpose, seeking the next pleasure – yet deep down I knew there was something more than simply following the next available pleasure. I urge you to rethink your life, constantly, matter who you are, or what you've accomplished. Humble yourself and identify the discomforts and obstacles you can actively move towards.

One day I came to the realisation that life itself was is lived on the *other* side of discomfort.

Power which we gain through more capable bodies and minds is best spent in continued improvement, rather than boasting over success. We should spend our life preparing for changes, which will happen despite any accomplishment made. If we resist this urge and let success over-inflate our egos, we will inevitably experience the toxic nature of success. We may build up an incredible physique, but as our testosterone levels decline with age we become prone to injury. If your ego has invested your worth in your physical capabilities, then you have a self-fulfilling prophecy of impossible satisfaction. Your bones will become brittle, your muscles will weaken, but your will won't dissipate; resistance will always be there to push against you, despite what body you *had* or what you *did* accomplish. Resistance will always keep pushing against you as long as you live another day. Ask yourself: "Will I have anything left once my body becomes weak?"

Let us embrace the struggle that is life and welcome the difficulty. Embrace the agony training the body will bring and prosper in the beauty and strength that will arise from your discipline. Although knowledge is powerful, remember that it is in the proof of progress which others will celebrate. We must be doers rather than thinkers. If the body isn't able to deal appropriately with addictions and degenerative habits, life inevitably becomes "unfair" and victimising, a cause of melancholy.

As Stoics, we train our bodies and minds to be ready to meet life's unfairness. We do not wallow in our gluttony; we welcome and embrace these temptations as a fortunate opportunity to become better versions of ourselves.

The Stoics do not care if you are under 10 per cent body fat, or whether you can deadlift a weight so heavy it would categorise you as an "elite weightlifter". The Stoics couldn't care less if your abdominals are visible, or whether veins are protruding through your forearms. If you want to get a six-pack, that's up to you – but don't let a goal like that become your purpose. Use your self-control and discipline in physical training as a constant test and reminder of your fight through vice. Remember that everything that happens in life is as common as roses which flower in summer; likewise with disease, with hardship, and everything else that pleases the soul or vexes a man. In absolutely every condition of life there is possibility of finding amusement, pleasure and fondness of the little things – but this is impossible if you consistently complain, identity yourself as unfortunate and unlucky and, worst of all, if you embrace being a man ungrateful of his position in life, a self-labelled victim.

By leaning on the masters of the past who dedicated their life to reflecting on the complexity of life we can think about food in a philosophical sense, eating in a manner which is reasonable, ethical and moving the body in the correct way. Philosophy is such a powerful tool in our lives. Science is more important, but philosophy helps us do better science. With something as simple as food and exercise we can gain a wider understanding for mastery over our entire lives.

Remember, this isn't a book explicitly on how to be a Stoic. It's a book on how to take care of your health as a Stoic would in the modern world. Refer to the recommended reading section for some books exclusively on Stoic philosophy. Although you have likely come away with a fair amount of knowledge about the basics, there are other concepts, ideas and historical moments worth learning about. An example could be a more in-depth look at how other schools of philosophy (Epicureans, Academics, Cynics, Socrates and the Sceptics) influenced the evolution of Stoicism and the distinct views they held.

I have placed great emphasis on the ethics of Stoicism as actually *living* the philosophy. Let's call this "active knowledge". Epictetus' promise of philosophy was the idea that being pragmatic and practical with little knowledge about Stoicism is better than having a complete and detailed academic under-standing but then living through a paradigm of hedonism. As I said previously, many of us may spend too much frivolous time thinking about the meaning of life and pondering on these concepts when the answer we are looking for is right in front of us.

So here you are; you've finished the book. So what are you left with? Your choices and your time. I think it's wise for me to end with a quote, so here is one of my all-time favourites:

"People are frugal in guarding their personal property; but as soon as it comes to squandering time they are most wasteful of the one thing in which it is right to be stingy."

– Seneca

REFERENCES

- Alirezaei, M., Kemball, C. C., Flynn, C. T., Wood, M. R., Whitton, J. L., & Kiosses, W. B. (2010). Short-term fasting induces profound neuronal autophagy. Autophagy, 6(6), 702-710. doi:10.4161/auto.6.6.12376

- Anson, R. M., Guo, Z., Cabo, R. D., Iyun, T., Rios, M., Hagepanos, A., . . . Mattson, M. P. (2003). Intermittent fasting dissociates beneficial effects of dietary restriction on glucose metabolism and neuronal resistance to injury from calorie intake. Proceedings of the National Academy of Sciences, 100(10), 6216-6220. doi:10.1073/pnas.1035720100

- A Varady , K., & K Hellerstein, M. (2007). Alternate-day fasting and chronic disease prevention: a review of human and animal trials. Search Results The American Journal of Clinical Nutrition, 86, 7-12. Retrieved January 13, 2017.

- American Academy of Microbiology. (2010). Microbe Magazine, 5(6), 268-268. doi:10.1128/microbe.5.268.2

- Anderson, J. K. (1985). Hunting in the ancient world. Berkeley, CA: Univ. of California Pr.

- Antelmi, E., Vinai, P., Pizza, F., Marcatelli, M., Speciale, M., & Provini, F. (2014). Nocturnal eating is part of the clinical spectrum of restless legs syndrome and an underestimated risk factor for increased body mass index. Sleep Medicine, 15(2), 168-172. doi:10.1016/j.sleep.2013.08.796

- Bucher, C. A., & Wuest, D. A. (1995). Foundations of physical education and sport. Mosby.

- Bhupathiraju, S. N., Pan, A., Malik, V. S., Manson, J. E., Willett, W. C., Dam, R. M., & Hu, F. B. (2012). Caffeinated and caffeine-free beverages and risk of type 2 diabetes. American Journal of Clinical Nutrition, 97(1), 155-166. doi:10.3945/ajcn.112.048603

- Barnosky, A. R., Hoddy, K. K., Unterman, T. G., & Varady, K. A. (2014). Intermittent fasting vs daily calorie restriction for type 2 diabetes prevention: a review of human findings. Translational Research, 164(4), 302-311. doi:10.1016/j.trsl.2014.05.013

- Berbesque, J. C., Marlowe, F. W., Shaw, P., & Thompson, P. (2014). Hunter-gatherers have less famine than agriculturalists. Biology Letters, 10(1), 20130853-20130853. doi:10.1098/rsbl.2013.0853

- Bicchieri, M. G. (1972). Hunters and gatherers today.

- Brosse, A. L., Sheets, E. S., Lett, H. S., & Blumenthal, J. A. (2002). Exercise and the Treatment of Clinical Depression in Adults. Sports Medicine, 32(12), 741-760. doi:10.2165/00007256-200232120-00001

- Bray, G. A., Smith, S. R., Jonge, L. D., Xie, H., Rood, J., Martin, C. K., … Redman, L. M. (2012). Effect of Dietary Protein Content on Weight Gain, Energy Expenditure, and Body Composition During Overeating. Jama, 307(1), 47. doi:10.1001/jama.2011.1918

- Buijze, G. A., Sierevelt, I. N., Bas C. J. M. Van Der Heijden, Dijkgraaf, M. G., & Frings-Dresen, M. H. (2016). The Effect of Cold Showering on Health and Work: A Randomized Controlled Trial. Plos One, 11(9). doi:10.1371/journal.pone.0161749

- Barsh, G., Farooqi, I., & O'Rahilly, S. (2000). Genetics of body-weight regulation. Nature, 404(6778), 644-51. doi:10.1038/35007519

- Brenner, I., Castellani, J., Gabaree, C., Young, A., Zamecnik, J., Shephard, R., & Shek, P. (1999). Immune changes in humans during cold exposure: effects of prior heating and exercise. Journal of Applied Physiology, 87(2), 699-710. Retrieved May 22, 2017, from https://www.ncbi.nlm.nih.gov/pubmed/10444630.

- Cancello, R., Tounian, A., Poitou, C., & Clément, K. (2004). Adiposity signals, genetic and body weight regulation in humans. Diabetes & Metabolism, 30(3), 215-227. doi:10.1016/s1262-3636(07)70112-x

- Castillo, E. R., & Lieberman, D. E. (2015). Lower back pain. Evolution, Medicine, and Public Health, 2015(1), 2-3. doi:10.1093/emph/eou034

- Chanson, P., & Salenave, S. (2010). Metabolic Syndrome in Cushing's Syndrome. Neuroendocrinology, 92(1), 96-101. doi:10.1159/000314272

- Cicerón, M. T., Griffin, M. T., & Atkins, E. M. (1991). Cicero: on duties. Cambridge: Cambridge University Press.

- Castren, E., Voikar, V., & Rantamaki, T. (2007). Role of neurotrophic factors in depression. Current Opinion in Pharmacology, 7(1), 18-21. doi:10.1016/j.coph.2006.08.009

- Chandalia, M., Garg, A., Lutjohann, D., Bergmann, K. V., Grundy, S. M., & Brinkley, L. J. (2000). Beneficial Effects of High Dietary Fiber Intake in Patients with Type 2 Diabetes Mellitus. New England Journal of Medicine, 342(19), 1392-1398. doi:10.1056/nejm200005113421903

- Cotter, M. M., Loomis, D. A., Simpson, S. W., Latimer, B., & Hernandez, C. J. (2011). Human Evolution and Osteoporosis-Related Spinal Fractures. PLoS ONE, 6(10). doi:10.1371/journal.pone.0026658

- Colman, R. J., Anderson, R. M., Johnson, S. C., Kastman, E. K., Kosmatka, K. J., Beasley, T. M., . . . Weindruch,

R. (2009). Caloric Restriction Delays Disease Onset and Mortality in Rhesus Monkeys. Science, 325(5937), 201-204. doi:10.1126/science.1173635

- Challet, E. (2013). Circadian Clocks, Food Intake, and Metabolism. Progress in Molecular Biology and Translational Science Chronobiology: Biological Timing in Health and Disease, 105-135. doi:10.1016/b978-0-12-396971-2.00005-1

- Carlson, H., & Shah, J. (1989). Aspartame and its constituent amino acids: effects on prolactin, cortisol, growth hormone, insulin, and glucose in normal humans. The American Journal of Clinical Nutrition, 49(3), 427-32. Retrieved May 12, 2017, from https://www.ncbi.nlm.nih.gov/pubmed/2923074.

- Cabo, R. D. (2012). Impact of caloric restriction on health and survival in rhesus monkeys from the NIA study. Nature, 489(7415), 318-321. doi:10.1038/nature11432

- Coupé, B., Ishii, Y., Dietrich, M., Komatsu, M., Horvath, T., & Bouret, S. (2012). Loss of Autophagy in Pro-opiomelanocortin Neurons Perturbs Axon Growth and Causes Metabolic Dysregulation. Cell Metabolism, 15(2), 247-255. doi:10.1016/j.cmet.2011.12.016

- Czochanska, Z., Salmond, C., Davidson, F., & Prior, I. (1981). Cholesterol, coconuts, and diet on Polynesian atolls: a natural experiment: the Pukapuka and Tokelau island studies. The American Society for Clinical Nutrition, 34(8), 1552-1561. Retrieved September 12, 2017, from http://ajcn.nutrition.org/content/34/8/1552.short

- Crompton, R. H., Sellers, W. I., & Thorpe, S. K. (2010). Arboreality, terrestriality and bipedalism. Philosophical Transactions of the Royal Society B: Biological Sciences, 365(1556), 3301-3314. doi:10.1098/rstb.2010.0035

- Cypess, A. M., Lehman, S., Williams, G., Tal, I., Rodman, D., Goldfine, A. B., . . . Kahn, C. R. (2009). Identification and Importance of Brown Adipose Tissue in Adult Humans. New England Journal of Medicine, 360(15), 1509-1517. doi:10.1056/nejmoa0810780

- Davidson, R., & Lutz, A. (2008). Buddha's Brain: Neuroplasticity and Meditation [In the Spotlight]. IEEE Signal Processing Magazine, 25(1), 176-174. doi:10.1109/msp.2008.4431873

- Dandona, P., Ghanim, H., Chaudhuri, A., Dhindsa, S., & Kim, S. S. (2010). Macronutrient intake induces oxidative and inflammatory stress: potential relevance to atherosclerosis and insulin resistance. Experimental and Molecular Medicine, 42(4), 245. doi:10.3858/emm.2010.42.4.033

- Devettere, R. J. (2002). Introduction to virtue ethics: insights of the ancient Greeks. Washington, D.C.: Georgetown University Press.

- Davis, L. M., Pauly, J. R., Readnower, R. D., Rho, J. M., & Sullivan, P. G. (2008). Fasting is neuroprotective following traumatic brain injury. Journal of Neuro-science Research, 86(8), 1812-1822. doi:10.1002/jnr.21628

- Daubenmier, J., Kristeller, J., Hecht, F. M., Maninger, N., Kuwata, M., Jhaveri, K., . . . Epel, E. (2011). Mindfulness Intervention for Stress Eating to Reduce Cortisol and Abdominal Fat among Overweight and Obese Women: An Exploratory Randomized Controlled Study. Journal of Obesity, 2011, 1-13. doi:10.1155/2011/651936

- Duan, W., Guo, Z., Jiang, H., Ware, M., Li, X., & Mattson, M. P. (2003). Dietary restriction normalizes glucose metabolism and BDNF levels, slows disease progression, and increases survival in huntingtin mutant mice. Proceedings of the National Academy of Sciences, 100(5), 2911-2916. doi:10.1073/pnas.0536856100

- D., & Dorandi, T. (2013). Lives of eminent philosophers. Cambridge: Cambridge University Press.

- Eubulus. Semele or Dionysus, fr. 93. preserved in Athenaeus, Deipnosophists 2.37c

- E. (2009). Handbook of Epictetus. New York: ClassicBooksAmerica.

- Ekmekcioglu, C., & Touitou, Y. (2010). Chronobiological aspects of food intake and metabolism and their relevance on energy balance and weight regulation. Obesity Reviews, 12(1), 14-25. doi:10.1111/j.1467-789x.2010.00716.x

- Erdman, J., Oria, M., & Pillsbury, L. (2011). Nutrition and Traumatic Brain Injury. Institute of Medicine (US) Committee on Nutrition, Trauma, and the Brain. doi:10.17226/13121

- Erickson, K. I., Voss, M. W., Prakash, R. S., Basak, C., Szabo, A., Chaddock, L., . . . Kramer, A. F. (2011). Exercise training increases size of hippocampus and improves memory. Proceedings of the National Academy of Sciences, 108(7), 3017-3022. doi:10.1073/pnas.1015950108

- E., E., & Oldfather, W. A. (1966). The discourses. Cambridge, MA: Harvard University Press.

- Frias, J. (2002). Effects of acute alcohol intoxication on pituitary-gonadal axis hormones, pituitary-adrenal axis hormones, beta-endorphin and prolactin in human adults of both sexes. Alcohol and Alcoholism, 37(2), 169-173. doi:10.1093/alcalc/37.2.169

- Forgas, J. P. (2013). Don't Worry, Be Sad! On the Cognitive, Motivational, and Interpersonal Benefits of Negative Mood. Current Directions in Psychological Science, 22(3), 225-232. dos 10.1177/0963721412474458

- Fung, J. (2016). The obesity code: unlocking the secrets of weight loss. Vancouver: Greystone Books.

- Fichter, M. M., Pirke, K., & Holsboer, F. (1986). Weight loss causes neuroendocrine disturbances: experimental study in healthy starving subjects. Psychiatry Research, 17(1), 61-72. doi:10.1016/0165-1781(86)90042-9

- Fisher, R. A. (1930). The genetical theory of natural selection. doi:10.5962/bhl.title.27468

- Fraser, R., Ingram, M. C., Anderson, N. H., Morrison, C., Davies, E., & Connell, J. M. (1999). Cortisol Effects on Body Mass, Blood Pressure, and Cholesterol in the General Population. Hypertension, 33(6), 1364-1368. doi:10.1161/01.hyp.33.6.1364

- Fagherazzi, G., Vilier, A., Sartorelli, D. S., Lajous, M., Balkau, B., & Clavel-Chapelon, F. (2013). Consumption of artificially and sugar-sweetened beverages and incident type 2 diabetes in the Etude Epidemiologique aupres des femmes de la Mutuelle Generale de l'Education Nationale-European Prospective Investigation into Cancer and Nutrition cohort. American Journal of Clinical Nutrition, 97(3), 517-523. doi:10.3945/ajcn.112.050997

- Fowler, S. P., Williams, K., Resendez, R. G., Hunt, K. J., Hazuda, H. P., & Stern, M. P. (2008). Fueling the Obesity Epidemic? Artificially Sweetened Beverage Use and Long-term Weight Gain. Obesity, 16(8), 1894-1900. doi:10.1038/oby.2008.284

- Forbes, C. A. (1929). Greek physical education. New York: Century.

- Field, T., Diego, M., & Hernandez-Reif, M. (2010). Preterm infant massage therapy research: A review. Infant Behavior and Development, 33(2), 115-124. doi:10.1016/j.infbeh.2009.12.004

- Ferrieres, J. (2004). The French paradox: lessons for other countries. Heart, 90(1), 107-111. doi:10.1136/heart.90.1.107

- Guyenet, S. J. (2017). The hungry brain: outsmarting the instincts that make us overeat. New York: Flatiron Books.

- Garro, L. (1990). Culture, pain, and cancer. Journal of Palliative Care, 6, 34-44. Retrieved April 01, 2017, from https://www.ncbi.nlm.nih.gov/pubmed/2231198.

- Greenberg, J. A. (2013). The obesity paradox in the US population. American Journal of Clinical Nutrition, 97(6), 1195-1200. doi:10.3945/ajcn.112.045815

- Gallicchio, L., & Kalesan, B. (2009). Sleep duration and mortality: a systematic review and meta-analysis. Journal of Sleep Research, 18(2), 148-158. doi:10.1111/j.1365-2869.2008.00732.x

- Grant, M., & Huxley, G. (1964). The birth of western civilization: Greece and Rome. London: Thames and Hudson.

- Garnsey, P. (2002). Food and society in classical antiquity. Cambridge (U.K.): Cambridge University Press.

- Greenberg, J. A., & Geliebter, A. (2012). Coffee, Hunger, and Peptide YY. Journal of the American College of Nutrition, 31(3), 160-166. doi:10.1080/07315724.2012.10720023

- Habbu, A., Lakkis, N. M., & Dokainish, H. (2006). The Obesity Paradox: Fact or Fiction? The American Journal of Cardiology, 98(7), 944-948. doi:10.1016/j.amjcard.2006.04.039

- Halagappa, V. K., Guo, Z., Pearson, M., Matsuoka, Y., Cutler, R. G., Laferla, F. M., & Mattson, M. P. (2007). Intermittent fasting and caloric restriction ameliorate age-related behavioral deficits in the triple-transgenic mouse model of Alzheimer's disease. Neurobiology of Disease, 26(1), 212-220. doi:10.1016/j.nbd.2006.12.019

- Hadot, P., & Davidson, A. I. (2011). Philosophy as a way of life: spiritual exercises from Socrates to Foucault. Oxford: Blackwell.

- Hatori, M., Vollmers, C., Zarrinpar, A., Ditacchio, L., Bushong, E., Gill, S., . . . Panda, S. (2012). Time-Restricted Feeding without Reducing Caloric Intake Prevents Metabolic Diseases in Mice Fed a High-Fat Diet. Cell Metabolism, 15(6), 848-860. doi:10.1016/j.cmet.2012.04.019

- Horstmann, P., & Norman, J. (2001). Nietzsche: beyond good and evil. Cambridge: Cambridge University Press.

- Harris, H. A. (1989). Sport in Greece and Rome. Ithaca (N.Y.): Cornell University Press.

- Horne, J. (1989). Why we sleep: the functions of sleep in humans and other mammals. Oxford: Oxford University Press.

- Hatori, M., Vollmers, C., Zarrinpar, A., Ditacchio, L., Bushong, E., Gill, S., . . . Panda, S. (2012). Time-Restricted Feeding without Reducing Caloric Intake Prevents Metabolic Diseases in Mice Fed a High-Fat Diet. Cell Metabolism, 15(6), 848-860. doi:10.1016/j.cmet.2012.04.019

- Holiday, R. (2014). The obstacle is the way: the timeless art of turning trials into triumph. New York: Portfolio/Penguin.

- Hutcheson, F., Moore, J., & Moor, J. (2014). Meditations of the Emperor Marcus Aurelius Antoninus. Indianapolis: Liberty Fund, Incorporated.

- Harris, R. B. (1990). Role of set-point theory in regulation of body weight. The FASEB Journal, 4(15), 3310-8. Retrieved March 17, 2017, from http://www.fasebj.org/content/4/15/3310.abstract

- Hausswirth, C., Louis, J., Bieuzen, F., Pournot, H., Fournier, J., Filliard, J., & Brisswalter, J. (2011). Effects of Whole-Body Cryotherapy vs. Far-Infrared vs. Passive Modalities on Recovery from Exercise-Induced Muscle Damage in Highly-Trained Runners. PLoS ONE, 6(12). doi:10.1371/journal.pone.0027749

- Holiday, R. (2017). Ego is the Enemy: The Fight to Master Our Greatest Opponent. Sl.: Profile Books LTD.

- Irvine, W. B. (2009). A guide to the good life: the ancient art of Stoic joy. New York: Oxford University Press.

- Inwood, B. (2003). The Cambridge companion to the Stoics. Cambridge, U.K.: Cambridge University Press.

- Ihsan, M., Watson, G., Choo, H. C., Lewandowski, P., Papazzo, A., Cameron-Smith, D., & Abbiss, C. R. (2014). Postexercise Muscle Cooling Enhances Gene Expression of PGC-1α. Medicine & Science in Sports & Exercise, 46(10), 1900-1907. doi:10.1249/mss.0000000000000308

- Iwamoto, D. K., Cheng, A., Lee, C. S., Takamatsu, S., & Gordon, D. (2011). "Man-ing" up and getting drunk: The role of masculine norms, alcohol intoxication and alcohol-related problems among college men. Addictive Behaviors, 36(9), 906-911. doi:10.1016/j.addbeh.2011.04.005

- Johnson, H. (1989). Vintage: the story of wine. New York: Simon and Schuster.

- Joinson, A. N. (2008). Looking at, looking up or keeping up with people? Proceeding of the twenty-sixth annual CHI conference on Human factors in computing systems - CHI '08. doi:10.1145/1357054.1357213

- Janssen, S. A., Arntz, A., & Bouts, S. (1998). Anxiety and pain: epinephrine-induced hyperalgesia and attentional influences. Pain, 76(3), 309-316. doi:10.1016/s0304-3959(98)00060-8

- Jakubowicz, D., Barnea, M., Wainstein, J., & Froy, O. (2013). High Caloric intake at breakfast vs. dinner differentially influences weight loss of overweight and obese women. Obesity, 21(12), 2504-2512. doi:10.1002/oby.20460

- Kelly, E. B. (2016). The 101 most unusual diseases and disorders. Santa Barbara, CA: Greenwood, an imprint of ABC-CLIO, LLC.

- Kaati, G., Bygren, L. O., Pembrey, M., & Sjöström, M. (2007). Transgenerational response to nutrition, early life circumstances and longevity. European Journal of Human Genetics, 15(7), 784-790. doi:10.1038/sj.ejhg.5201832

- Kaufman, J. S., Asuzu, M. C., Mufunda, J., Forrester, T., Wilks, R., Luke, A., . . . Cooper, R. S. (1997). Relationship Between Blood Pressure and Body Mass Index in Lean Populations. Hypertension, 30(6), 1511-1516. doi:10.1161/01.hyp.30.6.1511

- Kratz, M., Baars, T., & Guyenet, S. (2012). The relationship between high-fat dairy consumption and obesity, cardiovascular, and metabolic disease. European Journal of Nutrition, 52(1), 1-24. doi:10.1007/s00394-012-0418-1

- Kenny, A. J. (2004). A new history of Western philosophy. Oxford: Oxford University Press.

- Kumar, S., & Kaur, G. (2013). Intermittent Fasting Dietary Restriction Regimen Negatively Influences Reproduction in Young Rats: A Study of Hypothal-amo-Hypophysial-Gonadal Axis. PLoS ONE, 8(1). doi:10.1371/journal.pone.0052416

- Katzeff, H. L., O'connell, M., Horton, E. S., Danforth, E., Young, J. B., & Landsberg, L. (1986). Metabolic studies in human obesity during overnutrition and undernutrition: Thermogenic and hormonal responses to norepinephrine. Metabolism, 35(2), 166-175. doi:10.1016/0026-0495(86)90119-8

- Keating, S. E., Johnson, N. A., Mielke, G. I., & Coombes, J. S. (2017). A systematic review and meta-analysis of interval training versus moderate-intensity continuous training on body adiposity. Obesity Reviews. doi:10.1111/obr.12536

- Kassam, A. (2016, July 03). Arctic Ramadan: fasting in land of midnight sun comes with a challenge. Retrieved May 17, 2017, from https://www.theguardian.com/world/2016/jul/03/ramadan-canada-arctic-fasting-hours-sunlight

- Leproult, R., Copinschi, G., & Van Cauter, E. (1997). Sleep Loss Results in an Elevation of Cortisol Levels the Next Evening. Sleep. doi:10.1093/sleep/20.10.865

- Liu, Y., Wheaton, A. G., Chapman, D. P., Cunningham, T. J., Lu, H., & Croft, J. B. (2016). Prevalence of Healthy Sleep Duration among Adults — United States, 2014. MMWR. Morbidity and Mortality Weekly Report, 65(6), 137-141. doi:10.15585/mmwr.mm6506a1

- Li, F., Liu, X., & Zhang, D. (2015). Fish consumption and risk of depression: a meta-analysis. Journal of Epidemiology and Community Health, 70(3), 299-304. doi:10.1136/jech-2015-206278

- Lovato, N., & Lack, L. (2010). The effects of napping on cognitive functioning. Progress in Brain Research, 155-166. doi:10.1016/b978-0-444-53702-7.00009-9

- Laertius, D., Yonge, C. D., & Seddon, K. (2007). A summary of stoic philosophy: Zeno of Citium in Diogenes Laertius book seven. England: Lulu.

- Long, A. A. (2004). Epictetus: a stoic and socratic guide to life. Oxford: Clarendon Press.

- Lesauter, J., Hoque, N., Weintraub, M., Pfaff, D. W., & Silver, R. (2009). Stomach ghrelin-secreting cells as food-entrainable circadian clocks. Proceedings of the National Academy of Sciences, 106(32), 13582-13587. doi:10.1073/pnas.0906426106

- Lenoir, M., Serre, F., Cantin, L., & Ahmed, S. H. (2007). Intense Sweetness Surpasses Cocaine Reward. PLoS ONE, 2(8). doi:10.1371/journal.pone.0000698

- Lazarus, R. S. (1966). Psychological stress and the coping process. New York: McGraw-Hill.

- Lopez-Garcia, E. (2008). The Relationship of Coffee Consumption with Mortality. Annals of Internal Medicine, 148(12), 904. doi:10.7326/0003-4819-148-12-200806170-00003

- Lackovic, V., Borecký, L., Vigas, M., & Rovenský, J. (1988). Activation of NK Cells in Subjects Exposed to Mild Hyper- or Hypothermic Load. Journal of Interferon Research, 8(3), 393-402. doi:10.1089/jir.1988.8.393

- Maridakis, V., O'Connor, P. J., Dudley, G. A., & Mccully, K. K. (2007). Caffeine Attenuates Delayed-Onset Muscle Pain and Force Loss Following Eccentric Exercise. The Journal of Pain, 8(3), 237-243. doi:10.1016/j.jpain.2006.08.006

- Motl, R. W., O'Connor, P. J., & Dishman, R. K. (2003). Effect of caffeine on perceptions of leg muscle pain during moderate intensity cycling exercise. The Journal of Pain, 4(6), 316-321. doi:10.1016/s1526-5900(03)00635-7

- Maroon, J. C., & Bost, J. W. (2006). ω-3 Fatty acids (fish oil) as an anti-inflammatory: an alternative to nonste-roidal anti-inflammatory drugs for discogenic pain. Surgical Neurology, 65(4), 326-331. doi:10.1016/j.surneu.2005.10.023

- Mooventhan, A., & Nivethitha, L. (2014). Scientific evidence-based effects of hydrotherapy on various systems of the body. North American Journal of Medical Sciences, 6(5), 199. doi:10.4103/1947-2714.132935

- Mckinnon, A. M. (2012). Metaphors in and for the Sociology of Religion: Towards a Theory after Nietzsche. Journal of Contemporary Religion, 27(2), 203-216. doi:10.1080/13537903.2012.675688

- Møller, S. E. (1991). Effect of Aspartame and Protein, Administered in Phenylalanine-Equivalent Doses, on Plasma Neutral Amino Acids, Aspartate, Insulin and Glucose in Man. Pharmacology & Toxicology, 68(5), 408-412. doi:10.1111/j.1600-0773.1991.tb01262.x

- Malaisse, W. J., Vanonderbergen, A., Louchami, K., Jijakli, H., & Malaisse-Lagae, F. (1998). Effects of Artificial Sweeteners on Insulin Release and Cationic Fluxes in Rat Pancreatic Islets. Cellular Signalling, 10(10), 727-733. doi:10.1016/s0898-6568(98)00017-5

- Mattison, J. A., Roth, G. S., Beasley, T. M., Tilmont, E. M., Handy, A. M., Herbert, R. L., . . .

- Mihrshahi, S., Ding, D., Gale, J., Allman-Farinelli, M., Banks, E., & Bauman, A. E. (2017). Vegetarian diet and all-cause mortality: Evidence from a large population-based Australian cohort - the 45 and Up Study. Preventive Medicine, 97, 1-7. doi:10.1016/j.ypmed.2016.12.044

- Moore, G. E., & Regan, T. (2003). The elements of ethics. Philadelphia, PA: Temple University Press.

- Montag, C., Markowetz, A., Blaszkiewicz, K., Andone, I., Lachmann, B., Sariyska, R., . . . Markett, S. (2017). Facebook usage on smartphones and gray matter volume of the nucleus accumbens. Behavioural Brain Research. doi:10.1016/j.bbr.2017.04.035

- Norem, J. K. (2008). Defensive Pessimism, Anxiety, and the Complexity of Evaluating Self-Regulation. Social and Personality Psychology Compass, 2(1), 121-134. doi:10.1111/j.1751-9004.2007.00053.x

- Neary, N., & Nieman, L. (2010). Adrenal insufficiency: etiology, diagnosis and treatment. Current Opinion in Endocrinology, Diabetes and Obesity, 17(3), 217-223. doi:10.1097/med.0b013e328338f608

- Oswald, I. (1980). Sleep as a Restorative Process: Human Clues. Progress in Brain Research, 53, 279-288. doi:10.1016/s0079-6123(08)60069-2

- Owen, N., Healy, G. N., Matthews, C. E., & Dunstan, D. W. (2010). Too Much Sitting. Exercise and Sport Sciences Reviews, 38(3), 105-113. doi:10.1097/jes.0b013e3181e373a2

- Östman, E., Granfeldt, Y., Persson, L., & Björck, I. (2005). Vinegar supplementation lowers glucose and insulin responses and increases satiety after a bread meal in healthy subjects. European Journal of Clinical Nutrition, 59(9), 983-988. doi:10.1038/sj.ejcn.1602197

- O'Keefe, J. H., Gheewala, N. M., & O'Keefe, J. O. (2008). Dietary Strategies for Improving Post-Prandial Glucose, Lipids, Inflammation, and Cardiovascular Health. Journal of the American College of Cardiology, 51(3), 249-255. doi:10.1016/j.jacc.2007.10.016

- Obesity and overweight. (2014). Retrieved April 07, 2017, from http://www.who.int/mediacentre/factsheets/fs311/en/

- Olivardia, R., Pope, H. G., & Hudson, J. I. (2000). Muscle Dysmorphia in Male Weightlifters: A Case-Control Study. American Journal of Psychiatry, 157(8), 1291-1296. doi:10.1176/appi.ajp.157.8.1291

- Overweight & Obesity Statistics | NIDDK. (n.d.). Retrieved April 22, 2017, from https://www.niddk.nih.gov/health-information/health-statistics/overweight-obesity

- Pilcher, J. J., Ginter, D. R., & Sadowsky, B. (1997). Sleep quality versus sleep quantity: Relationships between sleep and measures of health, well-being and sleepiness in college students. Journal of Psychosomatic Research, 42(6), 583-596. doi:10.1016/s0022-3999(97)00004-4

- Pigliucci, M. (2017). How to be a stoic: using ancient philosophy to live a modern life. NY, NY: Basic Books.

- Pinnock, C., O'brien, B., & Marshall, V. R. (1998). Older men's concerns about their urological health: a qualitative study. Australian and New Zealand Journal of Public Health, 22(3), 368-373. doi:10.1111/j.1467-842x.1998.tb01393.x

- Pejovic, S., Vgontzas, A. N., Basta, M., Tsaoussoglou, M., Zoumakis, E., Vgontzas, A., . . . Chrousos, G. P. (2010). Leptin and hunger levels in young healthy adults after one night of sleep loss. Journal of Sleep Research, 19(4), 552-558. doi:10.1111/j.1365-2869.2010.00844.x

- Publications, H. H. (2017, May 25). Supplements: A scorecard. Retrieved June 18, 2017, from http://www.health.harvard.edu/staying-healthy/supplements-a-scorecard

- Position of the American Dietetic Association: Vegetarian Diets. (2009). Journal of the American Dietetic Association, 109(7), 1266-1282. doi:10.1016/j.jada.2009.05.027

- Paoli, A. (2014). Ketogenic Diet for Obesity: Friend or Foe? International Journal of Environmental Research and Public Health, 11(2), 2092-2107. doi:10.3390/ijerph110202092

- Pasiakos, S. M., Cao, J. J., Margolis, L. M., Sauter, E. R., Whigham, L. D., Mcclung, J. P., . . . Young, A. J. (2013). Effects of high-protein diets on fat-free mass and muscle protein synthesis following weight loss: a randomized controlled trial. The FASEB Journal, 27(9), 3837-3847. doi:10.1096/fj.13-230227

- Plomp, K. A., Viðarsdóttir, U. S., Weston, D. A., Dobney, K., & Collard, M. (2015). The ancestral shape hypothesis: an evolutionary explanation for the occurrence of intervertebral disc herniation in humans. BMC Evolutionary Biology, 15(1). doi:10.1186/s12862-015-0336-y

- Mark, J. J. (2011, February 15). Zeno of Citium. Retrieved May 19, 2017, from http://www.ancient.eu/Zeno_of_Citium/

- Patrick, V. M., & Hagtvedt, H. (2012). "I Don't" versus "I Can't": When Empowered Refusal Motivates Goal-Directed Behavior. Journal of Consumer Research, 39(2), 371-381. doi:10.1086/663212

- Phillips, K. A. (2009). Understanding body dysmorphic disorder: an essential guide. Oxford: Oxford University Press.

- Panda, S., Hogenesch, J. B., & Kay, S. A. (2002). Circadian rhythms from flies to human. Nature, 417(6886), 329-335. doi:10.1038/417329a

- Redwine, L., Hauger, R. L., Gillin, J. C., & Irwin, M. (2000). Effects of Sleep and Sleep Deprivation on Interleukin-6, Growth Hormone, Cortisol, and Melatonin Levels in Humans1. The Journal of Clinical Endocrinology & Metabolism, 85(10), 3597-3603. doi:10.1210/jcem.85.10.6871

- Richards, T., & Hamilton, S. (2012). Obesity and Hyperbolic Discounting: An Experimental Analysis. Journal of Agricultural and Resource Economics, 37(2), 181-198. Retrieved from http://www.jstor.org/stable/23496707

- Roe, J., Thompson, C., Aspinall, P., Brewer, M., Duff, E., Miller, D., . . . Clow, A. (2013). Green Space and Stress: Evidence from Cortisol Measures in Deprived Urban Communities. International Journal of Environmental Research and Public Health, 10(9), 4086-4103. doi:10.3390/ijerph10094086

- Renwick, A. G., & Molinary, S. V. (2010). Sweet-taste receptors, low-energy sweeteners, glucose absorption and insulin release. British Journal of Nutrition, 104(10), 1415-1420. doi:10.1017/s0007114510002540

- Rosner, J. L. (2014). Ten Times More Microbial Cells than Body Cells in Humans? Microbe Magazine, 9(2), 47-47. doi:10.1128/microbe.9.47.2

- Rufus, C. M., King, C. A., & Irvine, W. B. (2011). Musonius Rufus: lectures & sayings. United States: Createspace.

- Riera, C. E., Tsaousidou, E., Halloran, J., Follett, P., Hahn, O., Pereira, M. M., . . . Dillin, A. (2017). The Sense of Smell Impacts Metabolic Health and Obesity. *Cell Metabolism, 26*(1). doi:10.1016/j.cmet.2017.06.015

- Ridaura, V. K., Faith, J. J., Rey, F. E., Cheng, J., Duncan, A. E., Kau, A. L., . . . Gordon, J. I. (2013). Gut Microbiota from Twins Discordant for Obesity Modulate Metabolism in Mice. Science, 341(6150), 1241214-1241214. doi:10.1126/science.1241214

- Savitz, J., Lucki, I., & Drevets, W. C. (2009). 5-HT1A receptor function in major depressive disorder. Progress in Neurobiology, 88(1), 17-31. doi:10.1016/j.pneurobio.2009.01.009

- Stimson, R. H., Johnstone, A. M., Homer, N. Z., Wake, D. J., Morton, N. M., Andrew, R., . . . Walker, B. R. (2007). Dietary Macronutrient Content Alters Cortisol Metabolism Independently of Body Weight Changes in Obese Men. The Journal of Clinical Endocrinology & Metabolism, 92(11), 4480-4484. doi:10.1210/jc.2007-0692

- Spengler, O. (2013). The decline of the West. S.l.: Stellar Books.

- Siri-Tarino, P. W., Sun, Q., Hu, F. B., & Krauss, R. M. (2010). Meta-analysis of prospective cohort studies evaluating the association of saturated fat with cardiovascular disease. American Journal of Clinical Nutrition, 91(3), 535-546. doi:10.3945/ajcn.2009.27725

- Schurgers, L. J., Geleijnse, J. M., Grobbee, D. E., Pols, H. A., Hofman, A., Witteman, J. C., & Vermeer, C. (1999). Nutritional Intake of Vitamins K1 (Phylloquinone) and K2 (Menaquinone) in The Netherlands. Journal of Nutritional & Environmental Medicine, 9(2), 115-122. doi:10.1080/13590849961717

- Sender, R., Fuchs, S., & Milo, R. (2016). Revised estimates for the number of human and bacteria cells in the body. doi:10.1101/036103

- Seneca, L. A., Stewart, A., & Seneca, L. A. (1900). Minor dialogues: together with the dialogue On clemency. London: G. Bell.

- S., & Campbell, R. (2014). Letters from a stoic: Epistulae morales ad Lucilium. London, England: Penguin Classics.

- Speakman, J. R. (2008). Thrifty genes for obesity, an attractive but flawed idea, and an alternative perspective: the 'drifty gene' hypothesis. International Journal of Obesity, 32(11), 1611-1617. doi:10.1038/ijo.2008.161

- Sarkola, T., & Eriksson, C. J. (2003). Testosterone Increases in Men After a Low Dose of Alcohol. Alcoholism: Clinical & Experimental Research, 27(4), 682-685. doi:10.1097/01.alc.0000060526.43976.68

- Sierksma, A., Sarkola, T., Eriksson, C. J., Gaag, M. S., Grobbee, D. E., & Hendriks, H. F. (2004). Effect of Moderate Alcohol Consumption on Plasma Dehydroepiandrosterone Sulfate, Testosterone, and Estradiol Levels in Middle-Aged Men and Postmenopausal Women: A Diet-Controlled Intervention Study. Alcoholism: Clinical and Experimental Research, 28(5), 780-785. doi:10.1097/01.alc.0000125356.70824.81

- Seneca, L. A., & Costa, C. D. (2005). On the shortness of life. New York: Penguin.

- Shapiro, H., & Curley, E. M. (1965). Hellenistic philosophy: selected readings in Epicureanism,

Stoicism, skepticism and Neoplatonism. New York: Modern Library.

- Solomon, R. L. (1980). The opponent-process theory of acquired motivation: The costs of pleasure and the benefits of pain. American Psychologist, 35(8), 691-712. doi:10.1037//0003-066x.35.8.691

- Sclafani, A., & Ackroff, K. (2012). Role of gut nutrient sensing in stimulating appetite and conditioning food preferences. *AJP: Regulatory, Integrative and Comparative Physiology,302*(10). doi:10.1152/ajpregu.00038.2012

- Schurgers, L. J., Geleijnse, J. M., Grobbee, D. E., Pols, H. A., Hofman, A., Witteman, J. C., & Vermeer, C. (2009). Nutritional Intake of Vitamins K1 (Phylloquinone) and K2 (Menaquinone) in The Netherlands. *Journal of Nutritional & Environmental Medicine, 9*(2), 115-122. doi:10.1080/13590849961717

- Stunkard, A. J. (1986). A twin study of human obesity. JAMA: The Journal of the American Medical Association, 256(1), 51-54. doi:10.1001/jama.256.1.51

- Scheer, F. A., Hilton, M. F., Mantzoros, C. S., & Shea, S. A. (2009). Adverse metabolic and cardiovascular consequences of circadian misalignment. Proceedings of the National Academy of Sciences, 106(11), 4453-4458. doi:10.1073/pnas.0808180106

- Tauchmanovà, L., Rossi, R., Biondi, B., Pulcrano, M., Nuzzo, V., Palmieri, E., . . . Lombardi, G. (2002). Patients with Subclinical Cushing's Syndrome due to Adrenal Adenoma Have Increased Cardiovascular Risk. The Journal of Clinical Endocrinology & Metabolism, 87(11), 4872-4878. doi:10.1210/jc.2001-011766

- Tilg, H., & Kaser, A. (2011). Gut microbiome, obesity, and metabolic dysfunction. Journal of Clinical Investigation, 121(6), 2126-2132. doi:10.1172/jci58109

- Thorning, T. K., Raben, A., Tholstrup, T., Soedamah-Muthu, S. S., Givens, I., & Astrup, A. (2016). Milk and dairy products: good or bad for human health? An assessment of the totality of scientific evidence. *Food & Nutrition Research, 60*(1), 32527. doi:10.3402/fnr.v60.32527

- Tong, J., Mannea, E., Aime, P., Pfluger, P. T., Yi, C., Castaneda, T. R., . . . Tschop, M. H. (2011). Ghrelin Enhances Olfactory Sensitivity and Exploratory Sniffing in Rodents and Humans. Journal of Neuroscience, 31(15), 5841-5846. doi:10.1523/jneurosci.5680-10.2011

- Varady, K. A. (2011). Intermittent versus daily calorie restriction: which diet regimen is more effective for weight loss? Obesity Reviews, 12(7). doi:10.1111/j.1467-789x.2011.00873.x

- Varady, K. A. (2012). Alternate Day Fasting: Effects on Body Weight and Chronic Disease Risk in Humans and Animals. Comparative Physiology of Fasting, Starvation, and Food Limitation, 395-408. doi:10.1007/978-3-642-29056-5_23

- Waters, T. R., & Dick, R. B. (2014). Evidence of Health Risks Associated with Prolonged Standing at Work and Intervention Effectiveness. Rehabilitation Nursing, 40(3), 148-165. doi:10.1002/rnj.166

- Wehr, T. A. (1992). In short photoperiods, human sleep is biphasic. Journal of Sleep Research, 1(2), 103-107. doi:10.1111/j.1365-2869.1992.tb00019.x

- Welsh, J. A., Sharma, A. J., Grellinger, L., & Vos, M. B. (2011). Consumption of added sugars is decreasing in the United States. American Journal of Clinical Nutrition, 94(3), 726-734. doi:10.3945/ajcn.111.018366

- Wells, J. C. (1990). Longman Pronunciation Dictionary. Harlow: Longman.

- Wells, S., Flynn, A., Tremblay, P. F., Dumas, T., Miller, P., & Graham, K. (2014). Linking Masculinity to Negative Drinking Consequences: The Mediating Roles of

Heavy Episodic Drinking and Alcohol Expectancies. Journal of Studies on Alcohol and Drugs, 75(3), 510-519. doi:10.15288/jsad.2014.75.510

- Wimbush, V. L., Byron, G. L., Valantasis, R., & Love, W. S. (2002). Asceticism. Oxford: Oxford university press.

- Wolf-Novak, L. C., Stagink, L. D., Brummel, M. C., Persoon, T. J., Filer, L., Bell, E. F., . . . Krause, W. L. (1990). Aspartame ingestion with and without carbohydrate in phenylketonuric and normal subjects: Effect on plasma concentrations of amino acids, glucose, and insulin. Metabolism, 39(4), 391-396. doi:10.1016/0026-0495(90)90254-a

- What's your beef? (2012). National Trust. Retrieved August 03, 2017, from https://animalwelfareapproved. us/wp-content/uploads/2012/05/067b-Whats-your-beef-full-report.pdf.

- Wing, R. R., & Hill, J. O. (2001). Successful Weight Loss Maintenance. Annual Review of Nutrition, 21(1), 323-341. doi:10.1146/annurev.nutr.21.1.323

- Wilson, E. R. (2014). The greatest empire: a life of Seneca. Oxford: Oxford University Press.

- Xenophon, .., Bonnette, A. L., & Bruell, C. J. (2014). Memorabilia. Ithaca: Cornell University Press.

- Zeller, E., & Reichel, O. J. (2013). The Stoics, Epicureans and Sceptics. Miami, FL: HardPress Publishing.

ACKNOWLEDGEMENTS

Some of the greatest minds in the world of science and philosophy both ancient and modern provided me with the knowledge and inspiration to bring together *The Stoic Body*. I am to take no credit for the brilliant work these people have spent their lives uncovering; I am merely a vessel for these ideas to reach your life through a unique perspective. I'd like to thank my family and friends for their continued support. I'd like to give a big thank you to the cafes around Wellington for the copious amounts of coffee which fuelled my furious typing on my keyboard and most importantly to you the reader, thank you, because without you, none of this would of been possible. I also find it important to acknowledge my position in life which has given me the time and opportunity to sit down and express my ideas and thoughts, a position many people who are far more intelligent and gifted I will ever be will never have the chance to do; for this I am grateful. I hope you enjoyed the book.

71408664R00167

Made in the USA
Columbia, SC
26 August 2019